GW01159427

SIRTFOOD DIET

Easy and Healthy Recipes for Weight Loss & Get Lean

(Burn Fat While Still Enjoying Your Favorite Foods)

Sonja Mair

Published by Alex Howard

© **Sonja Mair**

All Rights Reserved

Sirtfood Diet: Easy and Healthy Recipes for Weight Loss & Get Lean (Burn Fat While Still Enjoying Your Favorite Foods)

ISBN 978-1-77485-013-8

Legal & Disclaimer

The information contained in this book is not designed to replace or take the place of any form of medicine or professional medical advice. The information in this book has been provided for educational and entertainment purposes only.

Table of contents

Part 1

Chapter 1: What Is The Sirtfood Diet?

The Sirtfood diet is a nutritionally healthy diet composed of foods which are capable of turning on the genes of sirtuin (SIRT1). The SIRT1 genes which are activated by these foods increase the metabolic rate of your body, improve your muscle tone and improve overall health.

The proponents of the Sirtfood diet were the UK nutritionists, Aidan Goggins and Glen Matten. They laid out a plan to drink three green juices together with balanced Sirtfood meals to kick-start metabolism and lead healthy, disease-free lives.

Few things are infected as much as nutrition by fads, frauds, and quackery. As such, we can consider every new diet through a prism of balanced scepticism. The latest to generate news is the Sirtfood diet, which will assist with weight loss and other advantages such as "stimulating rejuvenation and cellular recovery" if we are to take arguments at face value.

This latest diet for the uninitiated is based on food consumption that may interact with a family of proteins known as sirtuin proteins, or SIRT1-SIRT7. Adding to the undoubted attraction of the diet is the fact that the best sources allegedly include red wine and chocolate, as well as citrus fruits, blueberries and kale. Calorie intake is limited during the first three days (1,000 calories per day) and consists of three Sirtfood green juices, plus a normal meal rich in "Sirtfoods" Intake of calories is increased on days four to seven (1,500 calories) and is composed of two juices and two meals. In addition, the recommendation is to eat a balanced diet rich in sirtuin foods, together with additional green juices. The meal plans also include prawns and salmon.

It sounds good – and sirtuins are actively active in a wide range of cellular processes including aging, growth, and circadian rhythm. The diet is also partially focused on limiting calories. The nutritionists behind this suggest the diet "influences the ability of the body to burn fat and enhances the metabolic system."

Sirtfood History

What is a sirtuin, and how does it relate to calorie restriction?

Sirtuins are a group of genes involved in the regulation of organisms' lifespans. There are genes used in housekeeping. To put it another way, they are responsible for cell repair and maintenance.

There are 7 of these in mammals: SIRT1-7. They control cellular energy, cell death, aging, inflammation and so on.

Early research showed that the calorie constraint (restricting intake by 60-70 percent of regular calorie intake) extended rodent life. A variety of species including primates have documented similar findings.

The association of increased sirtuins and extension of lifespan due to calorie restriction was one of the most important findings in these studies. Therefore sirtuin activation is associated with longevity, and thought to be a secret to the 'youth fountain.'

Also known as the 'skinny gene' is SIRT1, because it regulates fat storage and metabolism.

Scientists then began to look for dietary elements which might activate sirtuin. That is how they identified the Sirtfoods. These foods are felt to mimic the activity of fasting, calorie restriction and exercise, and thus can accelerate weight loss and promote health.

Decoded Diet

And what do we think about the diet? The reaction from a science point of view is: Very little. In response to changes in energy levels, sirtuins contribute to the regulation of the fat and glucose metabolism. Also, they could play a role in the effect of calorie restriction on ageing improvements. This may be through the influence of sirtuins on aerobic (or mitochondrial) metabolism, declining species of reactive oxygen (free radicals), and increasing antioxidant enzymes.

Research also suggests that transgenic mice with higher SIRT6 levels live significantly longer than wild-type mice, and that changes in SIRT6 expression may be relevant to the ageing of some human skin cells. Often gradual metazoan (yeast) aging has been seen in SIRT2.

It sounds impressive and the diet has some glowing reviews but none of this is compelling scientific evidence of the Sirtfood Diet having similar effects on real people. Assuming that laboratory research on mice, yeast, and human stem cells has any bearing on real-world health outcomes — tainted as they are by a multitude of confounding variables-would be a colossal over-extrapolation.

Is the Sirtfood Diet actually healthy for you?

If there appears to be a bit of a shortage of the diet's checklist of popular ingredients, you 're not alone — many health experts condemn the Sirtfood Diet for being overly restrictive. Beckerman says she never recommended the Sirtfood Diet to any of her clients because of its tight restrictions on calories. "While I applaud the Sirtfood Diet for promoting the consumption of real ingredients, I denounce it for promoting calorie restriction and unhealthy eating rules." Like many other diets that remove food groups from regular consumption, Beckerman says the Sirtfood Diet may indeed lead to "disordered eating" since it also blends elements from intermittent fasting plans into the mix.

McKenzie Caldwell, MPH, RDN, who specializes particularly in women's nutrition and dietary wellness during pregnancy, says the calorie counts associated with the diet are by far the worst quality. "1,000 calories per day are only suitable for children aged between 2 and 4 years," she says, citing current dietary guidelines distributed by the Mayo Clinic. "Not only is this not enough energy to support an adult body, it is not possible to fit into all the macro- and micronutrients an adult needs in that amount of food ... The diet can cause weight loss in the short term merely because of its caloric restriction."

However, most importantly, both nutrition experts agree that there is little to no clinical evidence to support the healthy diet for sustained weight loss. "There is simply no evidence to support the argument that the Sirtfood Diet would have a positive impact on balanced weight loss," says Beckerman. "The diet creators claim to have put participants on the diet at their own gym but this supposed anecdotal study was not published or validated by true researchers or scientists."

The science of losing weight

Doubtless for some people the diet will seem to work. But scientific proof of the successes of any diet is quite a different matter. Of course, the optimal research to determine the feasibility of a weight loss diet (or some other result, such as ageing) would require a reasonably large survey – representative of the demographic we 're interested in – and random distribution to a treatment or control group. Outcomes would then be monitored over an adequate period of time with strict control over confusing variables, such as other behaviors that may have a positive or negative impact on interest outcomes (smoking, examination, or exercise).

Methods such as self-reporting and memory would limit this study but would go some distance to explore the efficacy of this diet. However, research of this nature does not exist and therefore we should be careful when interpreting basic science-after all, human cells in a tissue culture dish are likely to react very differently to the cells in a living person.

Diet tipple: route one?

When we consider some of the specific claims, further doubt is cast over this diet. Losses of seven pounds in one week are unrealistic and are highly unlikely to reflect body fat changes. Dieters consume about 1000 kcal per day for the first three days-about 40-50 percent of what most people need. This will result in a rapid loss of glycogen from the skeletal muscle and the liver (a stored form of carbohydrate).

But we also store about 2.7 grams of water for every gram of stored glycogen, and the water is high. So we also lose accompanying water for all the lost glycogen-and hence weight. Additionally, very stringent diets are very difficult to obey and result in elevated appetite-stimulating hormones, such as ghrelin. Hence weight (glycogen and water) will return to normal if the urge to eat is gaining.

In fact it is difficult to adapt the experimental method to the study of diet. Often, placebo-controlled trials with any degree of ecological validity are not possible, and the health outcomes that we are often interested in playing out over many years make research design challenging. In comparison, experiments of large populations rely on remarkably simplistic and naïve forms of data collection, such as recollection and self-reporting, which yield extremely inaccurate results. Health work has a tough job against the environmental noise.

Is there a Fast Fix?

Regrettably not. Sensationalized headlines and often hyperbolic representation of scientific data lead to the seemingly endless controversy over what – and how much – we should eat, fueling our obsession with a "quick-fix" or miracle cure that is an endemic social problem in itself.

The Sirtfood diet should be consigned to the fad pile for the reasons outlined-at least from a scientific point of view. Based on the evidence we have, suggesting otherwise is at best spurious and at worst misleading and damaging to the genuine goals of a strategy for public health. The diet is unlikely to provide much gain to communities struggling with a diabetes crisis, lurking in the shadow of obesity. As others have pointed out very clearly, special diets do not work and dieting in general is not a solution for public health for societies where over half of adults are overweight.

The strongest approach at the moment is to incorporate long-term behavioural reform with political and environmental power, directed at increased physical exercise and a sort of deliberate control of what we consume. It's not a fast fix but it's going to work.

The key to weight loss is quite simple at its core: either create a calorie deficit by increasing your calorie burning through workouts or decreasing your calorie intake. But what if you can miss the diet and activate a "skinny gene" without the need for an extreme calorie restriction instead? That is The Sirtfood Diet's premise, written by nutrition experts Aidan Goggins and Glen Matten. They argue the way to do it is by sirtfoods.

Sirt foods are abundant in nutrients that cause a sirtuin called a so-called "skinny gene." According to Goggins and Matten, when an energy shortage is created after you limit calories, the "skinny gene" is activated. In 2003, sirtuins became interesting to the world of nutrition when researchers discovered that resveratrol, a compound found in red wine, had the same effect on life span as calorie restriction but was achieved without reducing intake.

The 39 participants lost an average of seven pounds in seven days in the 2015 pilot study (done by Goggins and Matten) measuring the potency of sirtuins. Those findings sound amazing, but understanding this is a limited sample size observed in a short period is crucial. Weight-loss critics have concerns about the high promises, too. "The claims made are very speculative and extrapolate from studies that focused mostly on simple organisms (such as yeast) at the cellular level. What happens at the cellular level does not necessarily translate into what happens at the macro level in the human body," says Adrienne Youdim, M.D., Center for Weight Loss and Nutrition at Beverly Hills, CA.

Chapter 2: Secrets Behind Adele's Incredible Weight-Loss

Adele is a global superstar with her incredible voice earning an Oscar, 15 Grammys and multiple world records. She 's clearly a successful woman and we all know that. The soulful singer, however, has been making headlines lately, not because of her uncompromising talent but because of her visible weight loss.

Her weight loss was first noticed on October 25 at the birthday bash of musician Drake last year, but it's her most recent social media post that has fans talking about. Making her first Instagram post in 2020 in which she thanked essential workers during the coronavirus pandemic – as well as expressing her good wishes for her birthday, fans were surprised at her weight loss. Adele once admitted to People Magazine in the past that she would refuse to work with someone who had a problem with her weight, saying: "But when I signed a deal, most of the industry understood that if anybody even dared to say: 'Lose weight,' they wouldn't work with me."

Adele is yet to disclose her weight loss officially, so she has simply no justification to do so. The fact of the matter is that Adele is a beautiful, talented woman, no matter how she looks and how much she weighs. Her weight loss pales compared to the other amazing things she's accomplished in her young life and it really shouldn't be framed as the most amazing thing she's done in recent memory. That said, they 're curious about how the star did it for the ones on a weight loss journey.

But first of all why is her profile so different?

Besides her stunning body, viewers even noted the singer's face looked a little odd as well.

Adele has lost volume and fat on her face as a result of her weight loss. As a result, her features have been more pronounced with a sharper and more chiseled look of her jaw and bone structure. In fact, it's obvious she's changed her diet because she appears to have a much healthier glow. The fact is, your skin is what you eat and when you eat a rich antioxidant nutrient-dense diet your skin will definitely be grateful for it.

Adele and her journey through weight loss

1. She is apparently following The Diet of Sirtfood

The seventh most Googled diet in 2019, it's clear there's a bit of buzz around The Sirtfood diet, and with Adele's weight loss, the buzz will surely grow.

Nutritionists Aidan Goggins and Glen Matten created the Sirtfood diet in the United Kingdom, after publishing a guide and a book on the recipe in 2016. The diet focuses on sirtuins, a group of seven proteins found in your body that help to regulate a variety of functions including cell death prevention, metabolism regulation, inflammation, and the aging process. The diet requires one to consume sirtuin-rich foods, known as sirt foods, in an effort to activate the sirtuins that will boost fat burning and accelerate metabolism.

What will I eat on the Sirtfood Diet?

The Sirtfood Diet promotes the consumption of foods containing Sirtuins, as stated. These Sirtfoods are healthy and nutrient dense to eat regularly. They cover:

Green Tea

Powdered cocoa

TURMIC

Kale Kale

Onions

Petersils

Broccoli sprouts

Blueberry

Olive oil-Oil

Olive olives

apples

Red grapes

Chocolate

Oily fish such as salmon, truces and mackerel

How does the Sirtfood Diet meal plan work?

The diet is split into two phases and whenever you feel you need a bit of a weight-loss boost, if you should.

Phase 1

This phase lasts seven days, and is divided up as well. You 're limited to a total of 1000 calories per day for the first 3 days. Your diet is composed of three green Sirtfood juices (including kale, arugula, parsley, celery, green apple, lemon juice, and green tea) and one Sirtfood meal. Miso-glazed tofu, the Sirtfood omelet or a shrimp stir-fry with buckwheat noodles can be a mean.

You'll then require two green juices and two daily meals for a total of 1,500 calories a day on days four through seven.

Phase one aims at jumping your weight loss (apparently, during phase one you are expected to lose 7 pounds). During this period, the diet does recommend that you stop exercising, or at least cut back on your usual fitness routine as you will not be taking in many calories.

Phase 2

The second period lasts two weeks, which is referred to as the repair phase. The aim is to promote consistent, safe, and achievable weight loss.

There is no calorie cap but during this process you are advised to eat three nutritious meals rich in Sirtfoods, as well as drink one green water. The meal recipes include berries soy yogurt, and stir-fried prawns with kale and buckwheat noodles.

You can continue with the Sirtfood diet once you're done with the phases, all you have to do is tweak your meals a bit and include as many syrtfoods as you can. Additionally, you 're advised to remain healthy after you've followed the Sirtfood lifestyle.

Okay but with the Sirtfood diet, can I lose weight?

Considering that you consume less calories than usual, yes, you are likely to lose weight by taking this diet. However, it's debatable if that particular approach is safe. This is because super-restrictive eating is rarely sustainable or healthy.

The Sirtfood Diet is healthy for me, then?

If you consider that 1,000 calories per day are only suitable for a child between the ages of 2 and 4, then I wouldn't call this diet plan healthy exactly. Yes, the diet may allow weight loss but it would be questionable to live on this kind of calorie restriction for too long.

Yeah, there's no telling that the Sirtfood diet foods are perfect for that. Lots of study has found that green tea, turmeric and even dark chocolate can provide the body with a variety of health benefits that include decreased risk of heart disease, diabetes and other inflammation-related diseases. But actual research into the long-term benefits of increased levels of sirtuin in humans is still in its early stages. On top of that, calorie control isn't how you want your life to be.

Yes, Adele looks awesome but if she follows the Sirtfood diet, she's more than likely tweaked it in a way that's sustainable and safer for her health. That being said, it's wise to reach out to a certified dietitian and get their thoughts. Our bodies are different from each other and following this particular diet doesn't mean you 're going to get Adele-results.

2. She enjoys Pilates, the Reformer

After being introduced to it by close friend Ayda Field, X Factor judge and singer Robbie Williams' wife, the singer took up Reformer Pilates according to the Daily Mail.

We all know that Pilates is a perfect workout for the body and for Reformer Pilates the same can be said. Reformer Pilates is a more technical version of regular Pilates that requires practitioners to use ropes, springs, and a carriage to move Pilates on special machines. The exercises include a full-body workout of high strength and low effects. Reformer Pilates helps improve posture, strength and flexibility and build a stronger core and muscle tone.

3. She specializes in being healthy and happy.

Adele has never shied away from being confident in her skin and herself. Although the star is known for her heart-wrenching ballads, self-love is obviously her highest priority. Adele celebrated her 31st birthday last year, and posted an Instagram post that proposed putting self-love first.

"I'm ready to feel the world around me for the first time in a decade, and look up for once. Be kind to yourself, people, we 're just human, we 're going slow, putting down your phone and laughing out at every opportunity, "she shared. "It's just trying to Just respect yourself, and I just learned that this is more than enough."

Especially during these times it can be hard to do, but self-love will do miracles for your wellbeing. Aside from making you happier, research published in the journal Health Psychology has found that self-love can help you make better health decisions.

What's more, a separate study published in the journal Psychological Science found that recently divorced individuals who were kinder to themselves were better off bouncing back in the months following the separation than those who regularly criticized themselves. Considering that the award-winning singer is going through a divorce at the moment, it's safe to say she 's definitely practicing a lot of self-love.

Chapter 3: Biochemistry And Enzymology Of Sirtuins

Sirtuins are highly conserved enzymes of NAD + dependent deacylase found in all life phylae. Genes that encode sirtuins are distributed as single genes in virtually all unicellular organisms, with well-characterized examples found in mycobacteria, eubacteria, and archaea. Sirtuin genes are also encoded in single-cell eukaryote genomes including yeast and protozoa. In eukaryotes, sirtuins are generally encoded by multiple genes, leading to distinctive isoforms, so the isoforms have developed differentiated cellular functions based on the subspecialization of a common catalytic activity. Sirtuins are developed to recognize the NAD+ substrate and react with lysine-activated peptide and protein substrates to the dinucleotide, resulting in deactivation. The sirtuins react as NAD + -dependent lysine deacetylases in the canonical sirtuine reaction. Sirtuins are present in mammals in 7 distinct isoforms, called SIRT1-7. For SIRT1-3 and more weakly for SIRT5-7, NAD + -dependent deacetylation activity has been determined. Diversification of human sirtuines was accompanied by compartmentalization of the organelles. In specific, sirtuins SIRT3, SIRT4 and SIRT5 are preferentially found in the mitochondrial compartment, while SIRT1, SIRT6 and SIRT7 are primarily nuclear compartments. The cytoplasmic compartment typically contains SIRT2. Such compartmentalization allows for multiple desires for the substrates and specific biological functions.

Comparisons of the sirtuin reactivity genome as well as functional analyses of sirtuins from phylogenetically diverse organisms indicate that the sirtuins have retained biochemical roles as deacylases uniformly. The most conserved part of sirtuin proteins is their catalytic machinery, embedded in the center of most known sequences, with C and N-terminal flanking sequences involved in targeting, trafficking, and protein-protein interaction. The catalytic domain includes a binding pocket to allow NAD+ recognition, and consists of a folded domain called a Rossman fold. The domain also contains a hydrophobic channel that can tolerate a residual of lysine. The active site is designed to assemble the carbonyl oxygen of an acylated lysine substratum and the alpha face of the anomeric carbon of the NAD+ portion of the nicotinamide riboside at a reactive geometry. This binding proximity accelerates the acyl-oxygen's chemical reaction with the anomeric carbon, resulting in cleavage of the nicotinamide bond, ADP-ribosyl-transfer to the acyl-oxygen and eventual deacylation. Although there have been some interesting exceptions to this general chemistry, such as ADPribosyl-transfer to protein substrates, and ADP-ribosylation of small nucleophiles, this chemistry has been documented to occur on sirtuins derived from various species including human, archaea, protozoan, and mycobacterial organisms.

Substrates to sirtuin

Extended studies and reviews are outside the reach of this chapter on the broad spectrum of human sirtuin substrates. These target lists show sirtuins interact with a number of protein substrates of various forms. Additional reviews which examined substrates of sirtuin can be found elsewhere. Among the sirtuin 's notable substrate targets are histones, which are extensively modified by cycles of acylation and deacylation in chromatin. This initially resulted in sirtuins being known as histone deacetylases, or HDACs. Through several years of study, however, it is readily obvious that the bulk of sirtuin substrates are in general not histones, but instead proteins such as transcriptional regulators and enzymatic proteins responsible for functional changes in cellular biology. The observation that some sirtuins are largely confined to cellular compartments where there are no histones has led to this nomenclature being completely reconsidered. More precisely, sirtuins are deacylases of lysine, or KDACs. It is still possible that NAD + -dependent deacetylation is the most described reaction of sirtuin enzymes. Some examples of non-acetyl substrates are however known. SIRT5 for example is capable of eliminating succinyl and glutaryl protein lysine modifications. SIRT6 is apparently capable of deactivating long-chain fatty acids, such as a tweaked myristol cation found on NFÿB. Evidence from crystallography suggests that SIRT5 and SIRT6 deacylate these lysine modified cations to NAD + -dependent deacetylation by similar mechanisms.

Mechanisms of SIRT1-7 Regulation

Transcriptional Sirtuine Regulation

Restrictions on calories or nutrients are known to extend the life span of several organisms. The involvement of sirtuins in regulating the pathways of nutrient sensing and the combination of sirtuin activity with a central metabolite, NAD+, have provided hints that sirtuins may extend the lifespan. Interestingly, the yeast-based prototype sirtuin, silent information regulator (Sir2), was identified to extend replicative lifespan within this microbe. In addition, the overexpression of Sir2 homologues extends the lifespan of Caenorhabditis elegans and Drosophila melanogaster in experimental organisms. While some debate has arisen on the belief that sirtuins are genes of longevity, it has solidified the basic idea that increased sirtuin homologues activity gives increase in lifespan.

In multiple studies, overexpression of mammalian sirtuin homologues is linked to health benefits ts. For instance, overexpression of SIRT6 causes extended lifespan of the mouse. Moveover, mammalian sirtuin expression is altered by the availability of nutrients. A caloric restriction diet of 40 percent induces increased levels of SIRT1 protein in multiple tissues, including in rats in the brain, adipose, kidney and liver. In humans subject to a 25 percent calorie restriction, the expression of SIRT1 increases by 113 percent in muscle tissue as shown by RT PCR. In 12.5 percent reduced calorie intake combined with 12.5 percent increased exercise energy expenditure, the levels of SIRT1 increased by 61 per cent. These human studies indicate a clear coupling of SIRT1 expression with nutritional abundance perturbation, linking transcription of SIRT1 to that stress. Increases in SIRT3 1 Biochemistry and enzymology of sirtuins 8 and SIRT5 expression in mice's liver mitochondria are also caused by caloric restriction. Similarly, exercise raises levels of SIRT1 mRNA in young physically inactive men's skeletal muscle, and SIRT3 protein in mice's triceps. On the opposite, unhealthy intake of nutrients such as a high-fat diet increases both mRNA and protein levels of SIRT1 in mice adipose while obesity lowers expression of SIRT1 mRNA in subcutaneous adipose tissue in humans.

It is crucial to understand the transcriptional regulatory mechanisms that act upstream of sirtuins in the light of emerging evidence for different sirtuin isoforms regulating different metabolic processes. SIRT1 is the sirtuin isoform most studied, and SIRT1 transcription is subject to complex regulatory

22

transcriptional inputs. The promoter sequence of SIRT1 has identified several transcriptional binding sites, and several of the transcription factors are involved in the modulation of apoptosis and the cell cycle. SIRT1 transcription, for example, is regulated by oxidative stress and damage to the DNA. Two functional p53-binding sites have been identified in the SIRT1 promoter regulatory region. P53 is a tumor suppressor and a transcription factor which responds to stress. The p53 is activated under normal energy status, exposing its binding DNA domain. The activated p53 is recruited to two p53-binding sites that are present within the SIRT1 promoter, resulting in SIRT1 gene expression repression. When energy is deprived, forkhead box O transcription factor 3a (FOXO3a) is translocated to the nucleus where it complexes and removes p53 from the SIRT1 promoter, thereby promoting transcription of the SIRT1 genes. Interestingly, p53 is a direct target to deacetylation with SIRT1. Deacetylated p53 is destabilized and inactivated, thus facilitating a transcription of SIRT1. A SIRT1 substrate target, namely endothelial NOS (eNOS), affects the p53 activity. SIRT1 deacetylates and turns eNOS on.

In endothelial cells, eNOS produces NO and encourages GTP to produce cGMP. High content of cGMP decreases level p53 and allows transcription by SIRT1. SIRT1 expression is also regulated by a transcriptional repressor, Hypermethylated in cancer 1

(HIC1). HIC1 forms a transcriptional repression complex with SIRT1 after DNA damage caused by the topoisomerase II etoposide inhibitor. This complex binds directly to the promoter SIRT1 and suppresses the transcription to SIRT1. HIC1 knockdown significantly increases the expression of SIRT1, which in turn leads to p53 deacetylation and inactivation, enabling cells to survive under DNA damage influence. HIC1 may also repress SIRT1 transcription by forming a complex with an E1A-binding protein (CtBP) carboxy terminal. As a redox sensor, heightened NADH levels activate CtBP. Activated CtBP is dimerized and is strongly affin with HIC1. Changes in the cellular redox status can change CtBP 's recruitment to SIRT1 promoter and thus regulate the expression of SIRT1. In specific, the caloric restriction decreases CtBP 's interaction with HIC1 thus facilitating transcription of SIRT1.

Regulation by NAD+ Metabolism Alterations

NAD + binding to their catalytic sites initiates the reaction of the sirtuins. Thus, a limiting factor of sirtuin activity may be the cellular NAD + availability. NAD + is responsible in cells for transferring electron equivalents for various metabolic reactions such as β-oxidation fatty acid, glycolysis, and the TCA process. In this position, NAD+ and its reduced form NADH, by direct integration into metabolic pathways, systematically regulate and organize metabolic reactions with additional inputs from various nutritional and environmental signals. Due to its importance in metabolic reactions, in the course of evolutionary time scales, the coupling of NAD + levels to sirtuin protein deacetylation activity may have acquired regulatory importance. Importantly, intracellular NAD+ levels are dynamic and subject to multiple biosynthetic influences including de 1 Biochemistry and Sirtuins 14 novo enzymology and nutritional inputs as well as salvage pathways. Dynamics are also coupled with several major NAD+ degrading pathways, including NAD+ consumer activities such as PARPs, sirtuins and NAD+ glycohydrolases such as CD38.

NAD + levels alter and are thought to control sirtuin activities through diverse mechanisms and steady-state perturbations. NAD + can be synthesized through multiple pathways, but a central mechanism appears to be regulating it. De novo biosynthesis of NAD+ can occur via the kynurenine pathway through the amino acid tryptophan catabolism. The main input for NAD + homeostasis appears, however, to be the NAD + rescue process. This pathway transforms NAM, the NAD + user by-product, back to NAD +. NAM-based nicotinamide mononucleotide (NMN) synthesis is done by the homodimeric enzyme phosphoribosyltransferase nicotinamide (NAMPT). NMN is then adenylated to regenerate NAD+ by the mononucleotide adenylyltransferases of nicotinamide / nicotinic acid (NMNAT1-3). Disruption of NAD + rescue pathways leads to decreased NAD

25

+ level control, which precipitates decrease in sirtuin activity. NAMPT is the speed-limiting enzyme in this pathway and NAMPT activity levels are key to setting the NAD + level.

NAMPT overexpression greatly raises NAD + levels in neurons and fi broblasts, while NMNAT, another enzyme's overexpression in the rescue process, does not modify cellular NAD+ levels. In addition, NAMPT over-expression has been shown to increase NAD+ cellular levels in cell models such as endothelial cells , lymphocytes and cardiomyocytes, suggesting that high NAMPT levels can induce biosynthesis by themselves. Consistently, the pharmacological use of NAMPT inhibitors significantly suppresses cellular NAD + levels, cementing the view that NAMPT is essential for NAD + level homeostatic control. Factors which affect NAD + homeostasis are associated with stress. AMPactivated protein kinase (AMPK), for example, is a major sensor of cellular energy status and regulates cellular NAD + level. Activated by nutrient deprivation and exercise, activation of AMPK causes cellular NAD + level to increase activity of SIRT1 and enable increased deacetylation of target proteins such as FOXOs and PGC-1α. Such activities promote higher energy consumption by β-oxidation of fatty acids and biogenesis of mitochondrials. While the whole mechanism of AMPK activity at NAD levels is still under study, it is done in part by controlling NAMPT expression. It is interesting to note that signaling molecules which activate AMPK converge on SIRT1 activity.

In adipocytes, for example, the fibroblast growth factor 21 (FGF21) activates AMPK in a serine / threonine kinase 11 (STK11 / LKB1) -dependent manner and in turn induces SIRT1 activities. Recombinant FGF21 administration in ob / ob mice increases the level of phosphorylated AMPK in the white adipose tissue. Concomitantly enhanced PGC-1α deacetylation SIRT1 causes increased oxidative capacity of the mitochondrial and reduced body weight in these mice. Adiponectin has analogous Y. Yang, A.A. Sauve the myocyte effect 15. Binding adiponectin to its receptor will induce an influx of calcium which activates the kinase kinase β (CaMKKβ) protein dependent on calcium / calmodulin. CaMKKβ then activates AMPK to increase the activity of SIRT1 deacetylation on the PGC-1α. As a result adiponectin stimulates mitochondrial biogenesis in the skeletal muscle. Cellular NAD + level can also be increased by inhibiting NAD + enzyme intake such as poly(ADP-ribose) polymerase-1 (PARP-1). PARP-1 is an important cell consumer of NAD +. PARP-1 binds to the damaged sequence after identification of defective or dysfunctional DNA, and uses NAD+ as a substratum to pass poly(ADPribose) to acceptors like itself. High fat diet in mice shows a robust increase in PARP-1 protein levels and activity in the brown adipose tissue and muscle, while PARP-1 enzyme activity in these tissues has been reduced by fasting. It has been shown that PARP-1 knockdown or pharmacological inhibition raises intracellular NAD+ levels while increasing in vitro SIRT1 function. In their skeletal muscle and brown adipose tissue (BAT), PARP-1 −/− mice showed higher NAD+ content and SIRT1 activity. In these tissues also the mitochondrial activities have been improved.

Thus, PARP-1 activity inhibition can potentially be developed as a therapeutic strategy to improve NAD + levels in key metabolic tissues. NAD+ level effects on sirtuin activity, specifically SIRT1 and SIRT3, are consistent with the view that NAD+ is a positive sirtuin activity stimulating regulator. For example, Auwerx and colleagues have shown that genetic NAD + level upregulation in knockouts of PARP1 improves SIRT1 activity. This genetic manipulation increases biogenesis of mitochondria, resistance to toxicity caused by a high fat diet and provides sensitization to insulin. In a supplementary study, Auwerx and colleagues used the compound nicotinamide riboside (NR) to increase NAD + levels in tissue. This has resulted in improved insulin sensitivity, increased exercise endurance and improved resistance to high fat diet toxicity. Tissue blots of the proteins revealed reductions in FOXO1 and PGC1α acetylation, consistent with SIRT1 activation. Similarly, increases in SIRT3 activity were inferred from decreased SOD2 acetylation. Most recently, Brown and colleagues have shown that NR supplementation by activation of SIRT3 increases protection from noise-induced hearing loss. Other labs have also found upregulated NAD+ synthesis leading to activation of the sirtuin. Shin Imai 's laboratory has shown that either NAMPT or its NMN derivative can activate the sirtuin and treat metabolic syndrome.

Chapter 4: Sirtuins And Aging

For a long time, aging was considered a passive decline in physiological function which eventually followed by death. Nonetheless, mean lifespan in Western cultures increased from around 60 years over the last century to over 80 years. Much of this change was largely due to safer conditions, because of cleaner drinking water , e.g. fewer infectious diseases. However, the growing information on aging's pathophysiology indicated that aging and age-related diseases could be averted. In addition, aged individual tissues are subjected to various stresses to cope with, including but not limited to DNA damage, insufficient nutrient sensing, protein deficiency and mitochondrial dysfunction. Caloric restriction (CR) is a physiological condition defined by a reduction in caloric intake of 20-50 percent while maintaining a proper micronutrient balance. CR remarkably changed many conditions in many species, including worms, bees, and mice, linked to ill health and increased life span. CR was also studied in non-human primates, and while the effect on longevity was inconclusive, possibly owing to laboratory configuration variations, the older monkeys on CR were usually in better health. Although intensive investigation is still underway into the mechanisms by which CR achieves these better profiles, several metabolic signaling pathways, including sirtuins, were involved.

The C is marked with. In the early 1990s, elegans gene daf-2 (insulin / IGF-1 receptor homologue) as an aging gene based further attention on the molecular underpinning of age-related physiological decline. Indeed, it has identified extensive molecular networks that impinge on the aging process. Regulation of excess food receptors, such as insulin / IGF-1 or mTOR, reduces the longevity of life. Conversely, activating pathways related to energy deprivation, such as AMPK, sirtuins, or FOXO, extends lifespan.

Sirtuins in Lower Organisms as Aging Genes

After the discovery that a complex consisting of yeast Sir2p, Sir3p, and Sir4p regulates lifespan, the sirtuin field was first linked to ageing. Deletion of any of those genes resulted in shorter lifespan. This was due, in the case of sir3 and sir4, to the fact that both types of mating were expressed, resulting in sterility. That was not valid for sir2, however. Regardless of the type of mating, sir2-deficient yeast cells lived shorter than controls associated with the accumulation of extrachromosomal rDNA circles, a cause of replicative yeast lifespan. However, most convincingly, sir2's ectopic expression increased its lifespan by around 25%. Additionally, the yeast SIR2 gene proved critical

31

for the lifespan extension caused by CR. The role of the sirtuin genes in longevity was translated into other species following these initial discoveries. The C.C. The genome of elegans contains four sirtuin genes, sir2.1-sir2.4. Sir-2.1 is most homologous to Sir2p's yeast and similar to Sir2p 's extended nematode overexpression lifespan. The D y fl. Melanogaster has five homologues for sirtuin and dSir2 increases the lifetime when over-expressed as well. Those findings, however, were challenged and attributed to poorly controlled genetic background. Indeed, the lifespan extension was lost when the transgenic worms and flies were crossed back to identical backgrounds, although a small but significant effect may still be attributed to sir-2.1 overexpression in C. Elegant people. Although there is debate about the role of sirtuin genes in extending lifespan, there is considerable evidence that sirtuins are involved in managing normal health or protecting against stress conditions. SIR2 / sir-2.1 was most notably described as a crucial regulator of the CR-induced nutritional stress. Indeed, yeast did not show the beneficial effects of this dietary action when SIR2 was deleted, although similar results occurred in Sir2 -deficient flies. Worms with a lack of sir-2.1 did not survive longer on CR and demonstrated reduced lifetime when exposed to hydrogen peroxide, heat stress, or UV. In addition, and as discussed in greater detail below, C. Cantó, R.H. Houtkooper 215 activation of sirtuins using pharmacological agents, e.g.

resveratrol or NAD + precursors, prevents both mice and worms from multiple forms of pain, and increases worm lifetime.

Several groups embarked on the quest for pharmacological activators after SIR2 / sir-2.1 was identified as a metabolic regulator of CR and lifespan. Resveratrol, a polyphenol present in various foods like mulberries, peanuts and grapes, is the most popular example. Resveratrol, but also other polyphenols such as fisetin and butein, increased the activity of SIRT1 deacetylase against a target peptide labelled fluorescently, and increased the lifespan of yeast by 30–70%. Resveratrol also prolonged C lifespan. Elegans, D. Sir-2.1 / Sir2 melanogaster -dependent fashions. However, as with sirtuin overexpression, resveratrol 's effect on longevity in later research has been debated. In addition, several groups reported evidence that resveratrol may not activate SIRT1 in vivo directly, but rather through AMPK or PDE4 cAMP-degrading phosphodiesterase, although a direct allosteric effect on SIRT1 can not be ruled out.

As a result, SIRT1 small molecule activators were developed, resulting in a range of so-called SIRT1 activating compounds (STACs), most notably SRT1720. Although these compounds were substantially more potent than resveratrol with respect to SIRT1 activation in vitro, and some positive health effects were reported in mice (see below), no lifespan extension was found in simple organisms after therapy. A more recent sirtuin activation strategy is based on the premise that these enzymes require NAD+ as an enzymatic cosubstrate and that increasing NAD+ bioavailability determines sirtuin activity. To achieve this, two strategies have been developed either to increase the load of NAD + precursors or to block the use of NAD + by competing enzymes such as PARPs (poly(ADP-ribose) polymerases). Indeed, when worms were treated with NAD + Nicotinamide riboside (NR) precursor, or when NAD + consumption was blocked using PARP inhibitors, these worms lived 25 percent longer, an effect that was completely sir-2.1-dependent.

Sirtuins and Mammalian Aging

The evidence gained on lower eukaryote organisms raised the possibility that sirtuins could also influence the lifespan of mammals. The first complication to test such hypothesis is that seven sirtuin enzymes (SIRT1-7) are host to mammalians. Their initial characterization has already highlighted possible individual non-overlapping roles, as sirtuins may differ in city-specific subcellular compartmentalization, catalytic activity and substratum. Most studies have therefore focused on the possible role of individual sirtuins in ageing. In this context, only strong and definite connections between SIRT1, SIRT3, SIRT6 and ageing have been identified. We will therefore concentrate our attention on these three sirtuins.

SIRT 1

SIRT1 was early highlighted as a mammalian sirtuin that could influence the lifespan of the yeast Sir2 and worm sir2.1. In accordance with this, various experimental lines have shown how SIRT1 could be an attractive target for protecting against many ageing hallmarks. Mice overexpressing SIRT1 are protected from insulin resistance associated with age, osteoporosis, impaired wound healing and hepatic steatosis. Transgenic SIRT1 mice, however, do not live longer than wild-type mice. This suggests that over-expression of the whole body SIRT1 per se is not enough to improve the survival of mice, even if it prevents the onset of symptoms linked to aging.

At this point, why enhanced health span does not translate into longer lifespan would be questionable. Although this is not well known at the moment, one hypothesis is that SIRT1 overexpression in the late aging processes lacks linearity with SIRT1 activity, hence not endorsing healthspan forever. In line with this probability, NAD + levels, a co-substrate limiting factor for SIRT1, decrease significantly with aged. In fact, the levels of SIRT1 protein in tissues from old rats are higher than in young rats, but its activity is lower due to the reduction in NAD+. As a result, NAD + levels could also limit SIRT1 transgenesis' ability to maintain metabolic benefits in late aging phases. Alternatively, SIRT1 may protect against certain metabolic-related diseases, but may affect the animal's susceptibility to developing other primordial deathly diseases, such as lymphomas, or may even potentiate the incidence of PTEN-driven cancers.

Additional evidence on SIRT1 's role during aging comes from the use of SIRT1 activating compounds (STACs). While it is still controversial whether resveratrol activates SIRT1 directly in cellular contexts, resveratrol seems to need clear SIRT1 activity to promote many of its metabolic and health benefits in mammalian cells an organism. Resveratrol-treated mice don't live longer when fed regular chow diets. However, as observed in SIRT1 transgenic mice, resveratrol supplementation resulted in a marked decline in a variety of age-related effects, including retained muscle function, higher bone mineral density and decreased inflammation. Importantly, despite the similar lifespan on chow diet, resveratrol-fed mice were protected from lifespan reduction induced by high-calorie diets. Like resveratrol, SRT1720, a second-generation STAC treatment, also had protective effects against metabolic damage caused by high-fat feeding and increased insulin sensitivity, preventing lifespan curbing associated with high-caloric diets. However, the remarkable differences between the actions of resveratrol and SRT1720 are often clouded by equal questions about their mode of action. Furthermore, both compounds show substrate-specific effects on SIRT1 activity. While this may be somehow discouraging to extrapolate the effects of STACs solely to SIRT1 activation, it may, however, help to identify SIRT1 sub-sets of targets that could be key to regulating the health span.

One key point about using STACs or SIRT1 transgenic whole body mice is that they target activation in multiple tissues. This may not be the best strategy though. Calorie restriction, for example, has divergent effects in regulation of SIRT1 in the muscle and liver. Therefore, selective tissue-specific stimulation of SIRT1 could be important so that benefits of longevity are not blunted by compensatory benefits in other tissues where SIRT1 may be repressed normally during the aging cycle.

Recently it has been shown, in line with this concept, that brain-specific SIRT1 overexpression is sufficient to extend the lifespan and delay mice aging. The discovery that a second brain-specific c transgenic line did not display comparable lifespan effects led the authors to hypothesize that the lifespan impact of brain SIRT1 relies on an excellent equilibrium between expression rates of SIRT1 in the dorsomedial and lateral hypothalamic nuclei relative to other brain regions. To date, this is the only mammalian model of SIRT1 gain-of-function that shows increased lifespan.

Further information about how SIRT1 can affect mammalian lifespan can be obtained from faulty SIRT1 activity models. Total deletion of SIRT1 in inbred mice seriously damages embryonic growth and postnatal survival. SIRT1 deficient mice are viable when outbred, but metabolically unstable and often fail to survive the first year after birth. While CR generally extends lifespan in mice, preliminary data suggest that mortality in SIRT1-defective mice is rather exacerbated. A recent study has certified that the lack of SIRT1 in outbred mice hinders CR's ability to extend lifespan. Interestingly, heterozygous mice with SIRT1 showed similar CR lifespan extension than wild-type mice. This suggests that endogenous levels of SIRT1 are adequate to optimize the benefits of CR activated in lifespan.

The crucial function of SIRT1 in growth and early postnatal existence complicates the evaluation of SIRT1 's contribution to adult lifespan altogether. The use of temporally or spatially controlled models is therefore required to demonstrate the relevance of SIRT1 to the lifespan of adult mammalians. In order to overcome this issue, the Sinclair lab has recently generated a mouse model induced by tamoxifen that allows the SIRT1 gene to be temporarily deleted. The use of genetically modified mouse models to remove the tissue-specific SIRT1 gene has provided important evidence showing that SIRT1 is a central contributor to mammalian safety. Deletion of SIRT1 in the liver was commonly linked with hepatic steatosis, hyperlipidemia and other dyslipidemic-related complications, such as cholesterol gallstones. Similarly, removing SIRT1 in adipose tissue results in decreased adiposity and causes mice to develop obesity and resistance to insulin. In this regard , it is important to note that the deletion of SIRT1 in the muscle, a crucial tissue that contributes to the metabolic homeostasis, shows no overt phenotype.

Altogether, while the lifespan of these models has not been closely examined, most information to date indicates that SIRT1 is necessary for the maintenance of metabolic homeostasis and that defective SIRT1 activity leads to metabolic complications that could adversely affect lifespan.

Additional data on how SIRT1 can lead to mammalian lifespan can be derived from observations of genetic association in human populations. The results thus far,

However, the obvious correlation between SIRT1 and human longevity has not been underlined. Pioneering studies on German centenarians found no notable influence on exceptional human longevity by five known single nucleotide polymorphisms throughout the entire SIRT1 gene. Shortly afterward similar findings were published on a Japanese population and two more European-based reports. In none of these cases could associate

SIRT1 with higher prevalence in lifespan. However, this said SIRT1 targets, such as FOXO3a, were closely associated with increased longevity in humans. This may indicate that many of the observed effects of SIRT1 on mammalian lifespan may be secondary to protection against age-related diseases or by influencing lifespan effectors, such as FOXO3a, on activity.

SIRT3

SIRT3 was the first to establish a tangible connection between mammalian ageing and sirtuins. Human genetic studies indicated a link between SIRT3 polymorphisms and exceptional ageing even before its biological actions were elucidated. Concomitant efforts underlined how a polymorphism linked to an enhancer region of the SIRT3 gene could be clearly segregated in aged individuals, to the point where the allle lacking enhancer activity was virtually absent in males over 90 years of age. While further confirmation of such findings will be necessary, they suggest that reduced expression of SIRT3 could negatively affect longevity. A constellation of works has demonstrated how SIRT3 is a major mitochondrial deacetylase enzyme with key roles in maintaining mitochondrial function during the last five years. Because of the close connection between mitochondrial function and many age-related pathologies, it should not come as a surprise that SIRT3 may affect lifespan. While SIRT3 gain-of-function models have not yet been reported, the use of SIRT3 defi cient mice has shown that SIRT3 is critical to some of the caloric restriction's anti-aging effects, such as hearing loss protection. Additionally, SIRT3 deficient mice are vulnerable to insulin resistance growth and to worsen the metabolic damage done by high-fat diets. Strikingly, deletion of SIRT3 exclusively in the liver or muscle, given the drastic hyperacetylation of mitochondrial proteins in the corresponding tissues, did not result in any significant phenotype. This suggests (1) that mitochondrial hyperacetylation does not actually suggest mitochondrial dysfunction, and (2) that the health risks arising from global deletion of SIRT3 can not be clarified solely by abnormal SIRT3 expression in the liver or muscle tissue. Most of SIRT3's protective effects have been linked to SIRT3's ability to modulate the production and detoxification of reactive oxygen species (ROS) species. Consequently, SIRT3 acts may be assumed to have wider consequences for age-related pathologies that are significantly impaired by the metabolism of the ROS. In this respect, the links between SIRT3, ROS and aging were further consolidated when SIRT3 activity was also linked to oncogenic process protection

SIRT 6

While the most scientific attention has historically been given to type I sirtuins (SIRT1-3), recent reports highlight how SIRT6 could

41

actually take center stage in the relationship between sirtuins and mammalian ageing. SIRT6 deficient mice look fairly normal at birth but experience an abrupt degenerative phenotype, reminiscent of the progeroid syndrome, within a few weeks. This was followed by a serious hypoglycemia, which leads to one month of life to the death of SIRT6 null mice. Later efforts described SIRT6 as the Hypoxia Inducible Factor 1α (Hif1α) suppressor. Essentially, in the promoters of Hif1α and glycolytic genes, SIRT6 maintains deacetylation of H3K9 residues, keeping them in repressed state. Upon deletion of SIRT6, Hif1α is transcriptionally upregulated and generates an abnormal glucose uptake potential that results in severe hypoglycemia. Overall, this would highlight that SIRT6 will act as a vital metabolic regulator.

The latest discovery that transgenic overexpression of SIRT6 improves survival in male mice has further confirmed the effect of SIRT6 on mammalian lifespan. The lifespan extension encouraged by SIRT6 overexpression is however small, around 15 percent, and could not be due to avoidance of any age-related incident specific c. Instead, over-expression by SIRT6 simply delayed the aging process, with animals dying from the same spectrum of disease as wild-type mice. This observation was the culmination of several indirect evidence that the gain-of-function of SIRT6 could have an impact on the lifespan of mammals. First, it was demonstrated that SIRT6 overexpression prevents the metabolic damage and inflammation caused by high-fat diet. Second, SIRT6 was intimately associated with maintaining genomic stability. SIRT6 has recently been shown to serve as a suppressor of tumours. Hence, increased expression of SIRT6 during the aging process can be protective to delay physiological decline.

Many Backers

Unfortunately very little research on the functions of other sirtuins in the aging process has been recorded to date. Any possible linkage can be extrapolated only through very indirect evidence. There was no research, for example, about how SIRT2 gain-of-function affects longevity, and SIRT2 deficient mice have no apparent phenotype. However, several, but not all, studies have suggested that SIRT2 inhibition may be beneficial in the battle against neurodegenerative diseases, by decreasing neuron cholesterol levels. In contrast, SIRT2 was proposed to be cancer-protective, as SIRT2 is down-regulated in gliomas and gastric sarcomas, and inactivating mutations were found in melanomas.

So, speculating about a potential function for SIRT2 in tumor suppression would be enticing. All in all, these observations suggest that while SIRT2 's physiological influence on lifespan remains largely unexplored, SIRT2 's activity may be preventive against some ageing comorbidities.

SIRT4 and SIRT5 deficient mice still lack some overt phenotype and are indistinguishable from wild-type mice under basal conditions, SIRT5 mice also remain phenotypically indistinguishable from wild-type mice when confronted with a high-fat diet, however SIRT4 is shielded from body weight gain due to enhanced fat catabolism.

Until now, there are no human genetic studies demonstrating any association of ageing between the genes SIRT4 or SIRT5. However, the possible functions of the mitochondrial metabolism controlling SIRT4 and SIRT5 make it impossible to fully rule out the potential effects of these mitochondrial sirtuins in age-related disorders.

For eg, SIRT4 has been demonstrated to manage the balances between lipid synthesis and oxidation. SIRT4 suppresses the degradation of fatty acids thus encouraging lipid anabolism, possibly through deacetylation and suppression of malonyl-CoA decarboxylase (MCD).

This, in turn, would increase the intracellular amount of malonyl-CoA, which inhibits CPT1 activity allosterically, and thus the intake of lipids into the mitochondria for oxidation, while at the same time constituting a major backbone for lipid anabolism.

Moreover, SIRT4 was recently reported as a gatekeeper for glutamine metabolism, influencing the development of tumors in this way. All in all, SIRT4's complex metabolic actions make it difficult to predict any possible lifespan impact. In SIRT5, very little is known about onits physiological actions other than involvement in urea metabolism over prolonged periods of fasting.

Chapter 5: Fighting Fat And Losing Weight

Celeb gets weight loss. Celeb looks different and gets photographed. Fans are going wild and * dying * to know exactly how they were doing this. Coming in: Adele! The singer was spotted with a noticeably slimmer figure last year (and again on a recent holiday in Anguilla), and people are super curious about the eating plan she reportedly follows: the Sirtfood Diet.

While Adele has not spoken publicly about her weight loss, the New York Post claimed that by following the eating plan she lost 50 pounds (and her name was originally attached to the diet back in 2016).

The Sirtfood diet is said to be rich in foods containing a specific nutrient that helps to activate genes in the body related to fat loss and fat preservation (more on all this in a minute) Then other people say they enjoy it because there are some pretty good foods with these unique nutrients (wine and chocolate), and you don't feel cheated.

Some of the surprising results from our Sirtfood Diet pilot study wasn't just how much weight the participants lost, which was amazing enough — it was the amount of weight loss that most fascinated us. What attracted our eye was the fact that a lot of people lose weight without losing any muscle. In fact, seeing people gain muscle wasn't uncommon. This left us with an inevitable conclusion: fat had merely melted away.

Achieving a significant fat loss normally requires a considerable sacrifice, either severely reducing calories or engaging in superhuman exercise levels, or both. But contrary to that, our participants either maintained or lowered their level of exercise, and did not even report feeling especially hungry. In fact, some even struggled to eat all of the food they had been provided with.

How even that is possible? It is only when we understand what happens to our fat cells when there is increased sirtuin activity that we can begin to make sense of these remarkable results.

THE LEAN GENES

Mice that have been genetically bred to have elevated levels of SIRT1, the sirtuin gene that induces fat loss, are leaner and more metabolically active,1 whereas mice that lack SIRT1 are fatter and have more metabolic disease.2 As we look at humans, levels of SIRT1 have been shown to be slightly lower in obese people's body fat relative to their healthy-weight counterparts.3,4 In comparison, humans w have been shown to have lower levels of SIRT1.

Stack all that up and you begin to get a sense of just how important sirtuins are to decide whether we remain lean or get fat, and why you can produce such impressive outcomes by through sirtuin activity. This is because we get advantages on multiple levels through sirtuins, starting at the very root of everything: the genes that control weight gain.

To understand this better, we need to delve deeper into what is happening in our cells, which is causing us to gain some weight.

BUSTING FAT

We'll describe this in terms of a drug-ring film in Hollywood. The streets flooded with drugs is our body flooded with fat. The drug pushers on the street corners are the source to the weight gain peddling reactions in our heads. But in reality it's just the low-level thugs. The real villain is behind it all, masterminding the whole project, controlling any transaction that the peddlers make. This antagonist is referred to in our film as PPAR-π (peroxisome proliferator-activated receptor-ÿ). PPAR-ÿ orchestrates the cycle of fat production by flipping on the genes needed to continue synthesizing and processing fat.6 To avoid fat multiplication, you need to reduce supply. Stop PPAR-ÿ and you stop fat gain effectively.

Enter our hero SIRT1, who rises to bring the villain down. With the villain locked up securely, there's no one to pull the strings and the entire fat-gain organization crumbles. With PPAR-π 's operation stopped, SIRT1 is turning its focus to "cleaning the parks." Not only is this achieved by shutting down fat production and storage, as we have shown, but it is also altering our metabolism so that we continue to rid the body of excess fat. Like a successful crime-fighting hero, SIRT1 has a sidekick, known as PGC-1α, a central receptor in our cells. It effectively activates the development of what is known as mitochondria. Those are the tiny factories of energy that live within each of our cells — they drive the body. The more we have the mitochondria, the more we can produce the energy. But as well as encouraging more mitochondria, PGC-1α also urges them to burn fat as the fuel of choice to produce the electricity. Thus fat storage is blocked on the one hand, and fat burning on the other increases.

WAT or BAT, then?

We have looked thus far at the impact of SIRT1 on fat loss on a well-known fat form called white adipose tissue (WAT). That is the sort of fat that weight gain coincides with. It specializes in storage and expansion, is horribly stubborn, and secretes a host of inflammatory chemicals that resist fat burning and stimulate further accumulation of fat making us overweight and obese. That's why weight gain often starts slowly but is able to snowball so fast.

But the sirtuin story has another intriguing angle, involving a lesser-known type of fat, brown adipose tissue (BAT), which behaves quite differently. BAT is beneficial to us in complete contrast to white adipose tissue, and wants to get used up.

49

Brown adipose tissue really lets us conserve energy and has developed into mammals to allow them to dissipate vast quantities of heat-shaped fat. This is recognized as a thermogenic influence, and is important to helping small mammals live in cold temperatures. Babies also contain substantial quantities of brown adipose tissue in humans, but it declines shortly after birth, leaving smaller amounts in adults.

This is where activation of SIRT1 is doing something truly amazing. It changes genes in our white adipose tissue to transform and adopt the characteristics of brown adipose tissue in what is called a "browning effect. "8 This means that our fat reserves continue to function in a radically different way — instead of retaining energy, they start mobilizing it to be disposed of.

Sirtuin activation, as we can see, has potent direct action on fat cells, encouraging the fat to melt away. Even there, it's not over. The sirtuins also have a beneficial effect on the most important weight gain hormones. Activation of the sirtuin enhances insulin activity. This helps to reduce the insulin resistance — the inability of our cells to respond to insulin properly — which is heavily involved in weight gain. SIRT1 also enhances our thyroid hormones' release and activity, which share many overlapping roles in boosting our metabolism and ultimately the rate we burn fat at.

APPETITE CONTROL

There was one thing we couldn't wrap our heads around in our pilot study: the participants didn't really get hungry despite a reduction in calories. In fact, some people struggled to eat all of the food that was provided.

One of the big advantages of the Sirtfood Diet is that without the need for a long-term calorie restriction, we can achieve great benefits. The very first week of diet is the process of hyper-success, where we pair mild fasting with an excess of strong Sirtfoods for a double blow to weight. And we expected some reports of hunger here, as with all of the fasting regimens. But we've had absolutely none!

We found the answer, as we trawled through research. It's all due to the body 's foremost appetite-regulating hormone, leptin, nicknamed the "satiety hormone." When we eat, leptin increases, signaling the hypothalamus inhibiting hunger to a part of the brain. Conversely, leptin signaling to the brain decreases when we fast, which makes us feel hungry.

Leptin is so effective in controlling appetite that early expectations were it could be used as a "silver bullet" for combating obesity. But that dream was shattered by the realization that the metabolic dysfunction occurring in obesity actually causes leptin to stop properly working. In obesity, the amount of leptin that can enter the brain is not only reduced but

51

the hypothalamus also becomes desensitized to its actions. This is known as leptin resistance: there is leptin but it doesn't work properly any more. Thus, for many overweight individuals, the brain continues to think they are underfed even though they eat enough, and signals for them to continue to seek food.

The consequence of this is that while the amount of leptin in the blood is necessary to control appetite, how much of it enters the brain and can have an effect on the hypothalamus is much more relevant. It is here that the Sirtfoods shine.

New evidence shows that the nutrients found in Sirtfoods have unique advantages in reversing leptin resistance.11,12 This is by both increasing leptin transport to the brain and increasing the hypothalamus' sensitivity to leptin actions. So back to our original question: Why don't the Sirtfood Diet make people feel hungry? Despite a drop in blood leptin levels during the mild fast, which would normally increase hunger, adding Sirtfoods into the diet makes leptin signals more efficient, leading to better regulation of appetite.

As we'll see later, Sirtfoods also has powerful effects on our taste centers, meaning we get a lot more pleasure and satisfaction from our food and therefore don't fall into the overeating trap to feel happy.

Sirtuins are expected to be a whole new term for only the most committed dietitians. But hitting the sirtuins, our metabolism 's master regulators, is the foundation of any effective weight-loss diet. Tragically, the very nature of our modern society, with abundant food and sedentary lifestyles, creates a perfect storm to shut down our sirtuin activity, and we see all around us the consequences of this.

The good news is that we now know what sirtuins are, how fat accumulation is managed and how fat burning is encouraged, and most importantly, how to turn them on. And with this revolutionary breakthrough, the answer to effective and sustained weight loss is ultimately yours to take.

As we now learn, weight loss with conventional diet comes from both fat loss and muscle loss, and thus we see a pronounced decrease in the metabolic rate. This induces the body to regain weight once more normal eating habits are resumed. But holding your muscle mass with Sirtfoods keeps you burning more fat with a minimal drop in metabolic rate. This provides the perfect basis for weight-loss success over the long term.

In addition, muscle mass and function are predictors of well-being and healthy aging, and maintaining the muscle prevents the development of chronic diseases such as diabetes and osteoporosis and keeps us mobile into older age. Importantly, it also seems to keep us happier, with scientists suggesting that even the way sirtuins maintain muscle has advantages for stress-related disorders, including depression reduction.

All and all, weight loss when maintaining the body is a biggie, and an even more desirable outcome. It's a unique feature of the Sirtfood Diet and we need to get back to the sirtuins and their powerful effects on the muscle to better understand that.

Chapter 6: Recipes

Few important notes surrounding these recettes:

• Recipes mention Thai (also known as bird's-eye chilies) chilies. They are notably hotter than regular chilies if you've never had them before. If you are not used to spicy food, we suggest that you start with a milder chili such as serrano, which will adapt the amount to suit your taste. As you get more accustomed to having chilies daily in your diet, you may find that you are beginning to love hotter varieties so please feel free to try.

• Miso is a delicious fermented soybean paste packed in flavour. It comes in a variety of colours, typically white , yellow, red, and brown. The sweeter miso pastes are lighter in color than the dark ones, which can be quite salty. Brown or red miso will work well for our recipes but experiment with it by all means and see which flavor you prefer. Red miso seems to be the saltier of these, so you would prefer to use a little less of it if you go for this one. Miso 's flavor and saltiness can also vary from brand to brand, so the best bet would be to check which type you buy and adjust the amount you use accordingly, so it isn't too overpowering. That means a bit of trial and error, but eventually you'll get the hang of it.

• That couldn't be simpler if you haven't fried buckwheat before. We recommend that you wash the buckwheat thoroughly in a sieve first before placing it in a saucepan of boiling water. Cooking times can differ so test the kit directions.

• It will be better for all the dishes to have flat-leaf parsley, but if you can't get hold of it, curly it does.

• Onions, garlic , and ginger shall always be peeled unless stated otherwise.

• These dishes do not use salt and pepper, but feel free to season with sea salt and black pepper to match your own taste preferences. Sirtfoods offer so much flavour, you'll probably find that you don't need as much as you normally do. It is highly recommended to add black pepper to any dish that contains turmeric, as this will help increase the absorption of its key sirtuin-activating nutrient, curcumin.

Stir-Fry Asian Shrimp With Buckwheat Noodles

SERVICE 1

1/3 pound (150 g) raw jumbo shrimp shelled, deveined

2 Teaspoons of tamari (or soy sauce, unless gluten is avoided)

2 Extra virgin olive oil Teaspoons

3 ounces (75 g) soba (nodles of buckwheat)

2 Cloves of garlic, finely chopped

1 Thai chili, finely chopped

1 Teaspoon of fresh ginger, finely chopped

1/8 cup (20 g) raw, sliced onion

1/2 cup (45 g) of celery with leaves, trimmed and sliced, and leaves set aside

1/2 cup (75 g) chopped green beans

Cup 3/4 (50 g) kale, about chopped

Chicken stock 1⁄2 cup (100ml)

Heat a frying pan over high heat, then cook the shrimp for 2 to 3 minutes in 1 teaspoon tamari and 1 teaspoon oil. Load the shrimp into a tray. Wipe the pan out with a towel of paper, as you will be using it again.

Cook the noodles for 5 to 8 minutes in boiling water, or as indicated on the box. Drain and pack away.

Meanwhile, in the remaining tamari and oil over medium-high heat, fry the garlic, chili, ginger, red onion, celery (but not the leaves), green beans, and kale for 2-3 min. Add the stock and bring to a boil, then cook for a minute or two until cooked but crunchy.

Attach the shrimp, pasta, and leaves of celery to the pan, bring back to a boil, then remove and serve from fire.

Miso And Sesame In Ginger And Chili Stir-Fried Greens

SERVICE 1

1 Tablelitre Mirin

Miso paste: 31/2 teaspoons (20 g)

1 x 5-ounce (150 g) Firm tofu block

1 celery stalk (40 g), trimmed (about 1/3 cup when sliced)

1/4 cup (40 g) red, sliced onion

1 medium (120 g) zucchini (when cut, around 1 cup)

1 Chile Thai

2 Garlic Nails

1 Teaspoon of fresh ginger, finely chopped

Cup 3/4 (50 g) Kale, Cut

2 Sesame Seed Teaspoons

Buckwheat: 1/4 cup (35 g)

1 Teaspoon of turmeric powder

2 Extra virgin olive oil Teaspoons

1 Teaspoon tamari (or soy sauce, unless gluten is avoided)

Oven gas to 400oF (200oC). Line a small, parchment-paper roasting pan.

Mix both the mirin and the miso. Lengthwise cut the tofu, then diagonally split each slice into triangles in half. Cover the tofu with the miso mix and leave to marinate as the other ingredients are packed.

Slice the angle into the celery, red onion, and zucchini. Chop the chili, garlic and ginger thinly, then set aside.

Cook the Kale for 5 minutes in a steamer. Discard and set aside.

Place the tofu in the roasting pan, sprinkle the tofu with the sesame seeds and roast in the oven for 15 to 20 minutes until it has been nicely caramelised.

Wash the buckwheat in a sieve, then place it along with the turmeric in a saucepan of boiling water. Cook as directed by package, then drain.

Heat the oil in a frying pan; add the celery, onion, zucchini, chili, garlic and ginger and fry over high heat for 1 to 2 minutes, then reduce to medium heat for 3 to 4 minutes until the vegetables are cooked through, but are still crunchy. If the vegetables start sticking to the pan you may need to add a tablespoon of water. Add the tamari and kale, and cook for another minute.

Serve with the greens and buckwheat, when the tofu is ready.

Turkey Escalope With Sage, Capers, And Parsley And Spiced Cauliflower "Couscous"

Thin cutlets are ideal but there are two options to turn it into an escalope if you can just locate turkey breast. You should either use a meat tenderizer, a hammer or a rolling pin to pound the steak until it's around 1/4 inch (5 mm) thick, depending on how thick the breast is. Or, if you feel that the breast is too thick to work with, and you have a steady hand, cut the breast half horizontally and pound each piece with the tenderizer.

SERVES 1

Cauliflower: 11/2 cups (150 g), finely chopped

2 Cloves of garlic, finely chopped

1/4 cup (40 g) red, finely chopped onion

1 Thai chili, finely chopped

1 Teaspoon of fresh ginger, finely chopped

2 Spoonfuls of extra virgin olive oil

2 Tablespoons of turmeric soil

1/2 cup (30 g) of sun-dried, finely chopped tomatoes

1/4 cup (10 g) fresh, chopped parsley

1/3 pound (150 g) steak or turkey cutlet (see above)

1 Dried sage Teaspoon

1/4 Lemon Juice

1 Tablelit capers

Place the raw cauliflower in a food processor to make the "couscous" Pulse to finely chop the cauliflower in 2-second bursts until it resembles a couscous. Alternatively, you should use a razor, then finely cut it.

In 1 tablespoon of the butter, fry the garlic, red onion, chili and ginger until soft but not browned. Attach the cauliflower and turmeric, and simmer for 1 minute. Remove from heat and add the tomatoes that have been sun-dried, and half the parsley.

Coat the turkey escalope in the sage and a little oil, then fry in a frying pan over medium heat for 5 to 6 minutes using remaining oil, turning regularly. Add the lemon juice, remaining parsley, capers and 1 table spoon of water to the pan when cooked through. That will make a cauliflower sauce to serve.

Kale And Red Dal Onion With Bukkwheat

SERVICE 1

1 cup of extra virgin olive oil

1 Pound of mustard seeds

1/4 cup (40 g) red, finely chopped onion

2 Cloves of garlic, finely chopped

1 Teaspoon of fresh ginger, finely chopped

1 Thai chili, finely chopped

1 Teaspoon of mild curry powder (mean or warm, if you prefer)

2 Tablespoons of turmeric soil

11/4 cups of vegetable stock (300ml) or water

1/4 cup (40 g) dried, rinsed lentils

Cup 3/4 (50 g) Kale, Cut

31/2 pounds (50ml) of tinned coconut milk

Buckwheat: 1/3 cup (50 g)

Heat the oil over medium heat in a medium saucepan, and add the mustard seeds. When the mustard seeds begin popping, add the onion, garlic , ginger and chili. Cook until tender, for about 10 minutes.

Connect the turmeric curry powder and 1 tablespoon, then simmer the spices for a few minutes. Stir in the stock and bring to a boil. Add the lentils to the saucepan and simmer for another 25 to 30 minutes until the lentils are cooked through and a smooth dal is present.

Add milk to the kale and coconut and simmer for another 5 minutes.

In the meantime, cook the buckwheat with the remaining turmeric tablespoon, as per the box instructions. Drain alongside the dal, and serve.

Aromatic Chicken Breast With Kale And Red Onions And A Chili Salsa Tomato

SERVICE 1

1/4 pound (120 g) of skinless, boneless breast chicken

2 Tablespoons of turmeric soil

1/4 Lemon Juice

1 litre, extra virgin olive oil

Cup 3/4 (50 g) Kale, Cut

1/8 cup (20 g) raw, sliced onion

1 Teaspoon of fresh chopped ginger

Buckwheat: 1/3 cup (50 g)

TO THE SALSA

1 Medium sized tomato (130 g)

1 Thai chili, finely chopped

1 Mezzanine capers, finely chopped

2 Table cubits (5 g) of parsley, finely chopped

1/4 Lemon Juice

Remove the eye from the tomato to make the salsa, then slice it very good, making care to preserve as much of the liquid as possible. Mix with the chili, capers, lemon juice and parsley. You could bring it all in a blender but the end product is a little different.

Heat the oven to 220 ° C (425oF). In 1 teaspoon of turmeric, the lemon juice, and a little oil, marinate the chicken breast. Leave on for five to ten minutes.

Heat an oven-proof frying pan until hot, then add the marinated chicken and cook on each side for about a minute or so until pale golden, then move to the oven (set on a baking tray if your pan is not oven-proof) for 8 to 10 minutes or until cooked. Remove from the oven, cover with foil, then leave for 5 minutes to rest before serving.

Meanwhile, boil the kale for 5 minutes in a steamer. Fry the red onions and the ginger in a little oil, then add the cooked kale and fry for another minute until soft but not browned.

Cook the buckwheat with the remaining turmeric teaspoon, as per package instructions. Serve with chicken, vegetables, and salsa.

Harissa Baked Tofu With Cauliflower "Couscous"

SERVES 1

Red bell pepper: 3/8 cup (60 g)

1 Half Thai Chili

2 Garlic Nails

About 1 cubiccup extra virgin olive oil

Pinch of cumin to the ground

Pinch of coriander

1/4 Lemon Juice

Firm tofu 7 ounces (200 g)

Cauliflower: 13/4 cups (200 g), roughly chopped

1/4 cup (40 g) red, finely chopped onion

1 Teaspoon of fresh ginger, finely chopped

2 Tablespoons of turmeric soil

1/2 cup (30 g) of sun-dried, finely chopped tomatoes

1/2 cup (20 g) minced parsley

Oven gas to 400°F (200°C).

Slice the red pepper lengthwise around the core to make the harissa so you have nice flat slices, remove any seeds, then place the chili and one of the garlic cloves in a roasting pan. Add a little oil and the dried cumin and coriander and roast for 15 to 20 minutes in the oven until the peppers are soft but not too brown. (Leave the oven on at this setting.) Cold, then mix with the lemon juice into a food processor until smooth.

Lengthwise slice the tofu and then diagonally cut into triangles each half. Place in a small non-stick roasting pan or one lined with parchment paper, cover with harissa and roast for 20 minutes in the oven — the tofu should have absorbed the marinade and turned dark red.

Place the raw cauliflower in a food processor to make the "couscous" Pulse to finely chop the cauliflower in 2-second bursts until it resembles a couscous. Alternatively, you should use a razor, then finely cut it.

Thin out the remaining clove of garlic. In 1 teaspoon of oil, fry the garlic, red onion and ginger, until soft but not browned, then add the turmeric and cauliflower and cook for 1 minute.

Remove from heat and stir in the tomatoes and parsley, which are dried with sun. Serve with the tofu which is fried.

Muesli Sirt

You just add the dry ingredients and put the mixture in an airtight jar if you want to make this in bulk or cook it the night before. The next day all you have to do is add the strawberries and milk and it's ready to go.

SERVICE 1

Buckwheat flakes: 1/4 cup (20 g)

Buckwheat puffs: 2/3 cup (10 g)

3 Tablespoons (15 g) of coconut or dry cocoa flakes

Cup 1/4 (40 g) Medjool seeds, diced and pitted

1/8 cup (15 g), chopped walnuts

11/2 cups (10 g) of cocoa nibs

2/3 cup (100 g) hulled and chopped strawberries

Pure Greek yogurt (or vegan substitute, such as soy or coconut yogurt) 3/8 cup (100 g)

Mix all the ingredients together (leave off the strawberries and cream, if not instantly served).

Salmon Fillet Pan-Fried With Caramelized Endive, Arugula, And Celery Leaf Salad

SERVES 1

Petersil: 1/4 cup (10 g)

1/4 Lemon Juice

1 Tablelit capers

1 Clove of garlic, sliced roughly

1 litre, extra virgin olive oil

1/4 Avocado, stoned, peeled, and diced

Cherry tomatoes, 2/3 cup (100 g), half cut

1/8 cup (20 g) red, thinly sliced onion

13/4 ounces Arugula (50 g)

2 Spoonfuls (5 g) of celery leaves

1 x 5-ounce (150 g) fillet with skinless salmon

2 Spoonfuls of brown sugar

1 Endive arm, roughly 21/2 ounces (70 g), halved in length

Heat the oven to 220 ° C (425oF).

Place the parsley, lemon juice, capers, garlic, and 2 teaspoons of oil in a food processor or mixer for dressing and blend until smooth.

For the salad, combine the leaves of avocado, tomato, red onion, arugula, and celery.

Heat a frying casserole over high heat. Rub the salmon in a little oil and sear for a minute or two in the hot saucepan to caramelize the fish skin. Transfer to a baking tray and place in the oven for 5 to 6 minutes or until it is cooked; reduce the cooking time by 2 minutes if you like the pink served inside of your fish.

Wipe the frying pan out meanwhile and put it back on high fire. Mix the brown sugar with the remaining oil teaspoon and sprinkle it over the endive cut sides. Place the cut-sides of the endive in the hot pan and cook for 2 to 3 minutes until tender and beautifully caramelized. In the dressing, toss the salad and serve with salmon, and endive.

Tuscan Bean Stew

SERVES 1

1 litre, extra virgin olive oil

1/3 cup (50 g) red, finely chopped onion

1/4 cup (30 g) carrot, finely chopped and peeled

1/3 cup (30 g) celery, finely chopped and trimmed

2 Cloves of garlic, finely chopped

1/2 Thai, finely chopped chili (optional)

1 Herbs de Provence teaspoon

Vegetable stock: 7/8 cup (200ml)

1 x 14-unce (400 g) of Italian chopped tomatoes

1 Pureed Tomato Tablespoon

Drained weight: 3/4 cup (130 g) canned mixed beans

Cup 3/4 (50 g) kale, about chopped

1 Tablespoon of approximately chopped parsley

Buckwheat: 1/4 cup (40 g)

Place the oil over low to medium heat in a medium saucepan and fry the onion, carrot, celery, garlic, chili (if used) and herbs gently, until the onion is soft but not browned.

Stir in the collection, tomatoes and purée tomatoes and bring to a boil. Attach the beans and require to cook for 30 minutes.

Add the kale and simmer for another 5 to 10 minutes, then add the parsley, until tender.

Meanwhile, according to the box instructions, cook the buckwheat, rinse and then serve with the stew.

Strawberry Tabbouleh Bukkwheat

SERVICE 1

Buckwheat: 1/3 cup (50 g)

1 Tablespoon of turmeric soil

1/2 Cup Avocado (80 g)

Tomatoes: 3/8 cup (65 g)

1/8 cup red onion (20 g)

1/8 cup (25 g) dates Medjool, pitted

1 Tablelit capers

Petersil: 3/4 cup (30 g)

2/3 cup (100 g) hulled strawberries

1 litre, extra virgin olive oil

1/2 Lemon Juice

1 Ounce Arugula (30 g)

Cook the buckwheat with the turmeric as indicated on the box. Drain to cool, and set aside.

Chop the avocado, basil, red onion, dates, capers and parsley thinly and mix with the fresh buckwheat. Pick the strawberries, then mix the oil then lemon juice softly into the salad. Serve on an earthenware bed.

Baked Cod Miso-Marinated With Stir-Fried Greens And Sesame

SERVICE 1

31/2 cups of tea (20 g) miso

1 Tablelitre Mirin

1 litre, extra virgin olive oil

1 x 7-ounce (200 g) filet of skinless cod

1/8 cup (20 g) raw, sliced onion

Celery: 3/8 cup (40 g), sliced

2 Cloves of garlic, finely chopped

1 Thai chili, finely chopped

1 Teaspoon of fresh ginger, finely chopped

3/8 Cup Green Beans (60 g)

Cup 3/4 (50 g) kale, about chopped

1 Sesame seeds in tablespoon

2 Tablespoons (5 g) of parsley, chopped roughly

1 Tablespoon tamari (or soy sauce, unless gluten is avoided)

Buckwheat: 1/4 cup (40 g)

1 Teaspoon of turmeric powder

Mix the oil with the miso, mirin and 1 tablespoon. Rub the cod all over, and set for 30 minutes to marinate. Heat the oven to 220 ° C (425oF).

Bake the cod for about 10 minutes.

Meanwhile, heat the remaining oil to a large frying pan or wok. Stir-fry the onion for a few minutes, then add the celery, garlic, chili, ginger, green beans and kale. Toss and fry until the kale is cooked through and tender. To help the cooking process you might need to add a little water to the pan.

Cook the buckwheat along with the turmeric according to the packet instructions.

To the stir-fry add the sesame seeds, parsley, and tamari and serve with buckwheat and shrimp.

Soba (Buckwheat Noodles) In A Miso Broth With Tofu, Celery, And Kale

SERVES 1

3 ounces (75 g) soba (nodles of buckwheat)

1 litre, extra virgin olive oil

1/8 cup (20 g) raw, sliced onion

2 Cloves of garlic, finely chopped

1 Teaspoon of fresh ginger, finely chopped

11/4 cups (300ml) of vegetable stock, plus some extra if needed

13/4 spoonfuls (30 g) of miso paste

Cup 3/4 (50 g) kale, about chopped

1/2 cup (50 g) celery, chopped approximately

1 Sesame seeds in tablespoon

31/2 ounces (100 g) solid tofu, sliced into 1/4- to 1/2-inch cubes (0.5 to 1 cm) (about 3/8 cup)

1 Tablespoon tamari (optional, or soy sauce, unless gluten is avoided)

Place the noodles in a saucepan of boiling water and cook for 5 to 8 minutes or as directed on the pack.

In a saucepan, heat the oil; add the onions, garlic and ginger and fry in the oil over medium heat until soft, but not browned. Stir in stock and miso and bring to a boil.

Attach the kale and celery to the miso broth and simmer gently for 5 minutes (try not to boil the miso because you ruin the taste and make it textured grainy). As needed you may need to add a little more stock.

Add the cooked noodles and sesame seeds, and allow the tofu to warm up. If needed, serve in a bowl drizzled with some tamari.

Sirt Out Salad

SERVICE 1

13/4 ounces Arugula (50 g)

Endive the leaves 13/4 ounces (50 g)

31/2 ounces (100 g) of slices of smoked salmon

Avocado 1/2 cup (80 g), peeled, stoned and sliced

1/2 cup (50 g) celery, sliced with leaves

1/8 cup (20 g) raw, sliced onion

1/8 cups (15 g), sliced walnuts

1 Tablelit capers

1 Big Medjool date, chopped and pitted

1 litre, extra virgin olive oil

1/4 Lemon Juice

1/4 cup (10 g) chopped parsley

Place the leaves of salad on a tray, or in a large tub.

Mix all the remaining ingredients and serve over the leaves.

VALITIES

Substitute the smoked salmon with 11/3 cups (100 g) canned green lentils or cooked Le Puy lentils for a lentil Sirt super salad.

Replace the smoked salmon with a sliced fried chicken breast, for a chicken sirt super salad.

Simply substitute the smoked salmon with canned tuna for a tuna Sirt super salad (in water or butter, as preferred).

Char-Grilled Beef With A Red Wine Jus, Onion Rings, Garlic Kale And Potatoes Herb-Roasted

SERVICE 1

1/2 cup (100 g) of potatoes, peeled and cut into 2 cm (3/4) "diced pieces

1 litre, extra virgin olive oil

2 Table cubits (5 g) of parsley, finely chopped

1/3 cup (50 g) red onion, in rings

2 Ounces (50 g), sliced kale

2 Cloves of garlic, finely chopped

Tenderloin (about 11/2 inches or 3.5 cm thick) or sirloin steak (3/4 inches or 2 cm thick) 1 x 4- to 5-ounces (120 to 150 g)

3 Tablespoons red wine (40ml)

Beef stock: 5/8 cup (150ml)

1 Pureed Tomato Tablespoon

1 Teaspoon of corn flour, dissolved in 1 c.p. water

Heat the oven to 220 ° C (425oF).

Place the potatoes in a boiling water saucepan, bring them back to a boil and cook for 4 to 5 minutes, then drain. Place 1 teaspoon of oil in a roasting pan, and roast for 35 to 45 minutes in the hot oven. Switch the potatoes every 10 minutes to ensure cooking is all finished. Remove from the oven when cooked, sprinkle with the chopped parsley and stir well.

Fry the onion over medium heat in 1 teaspoon of the oil for 5 to 7 minutes, until it is soft and caramelized. Keep on dry.

Steam the kale for two to three minutes, then drain. Gently fry the garlic in 1/2 teaspoon of oil for 1 minute, until browned but not soft. Attach the kale and fry for another 1 to 2 minutes, before tender. Keep on dry.

Heat up a frying pan which is ovenproof over high heat until smoking. Coat the meat with 1/2 teaspoon of the oil and fry over medium-high heat in the hot pan, depending on how you like your meat (see our cooking times guide). If you like your meat medium, it would be better to sear it and then transfer it to an oven set at 425oF (220oC) for the prescribed times.

Remove the meat from the saucepan and set to rest. To bring up any meat residue add the wine to the hot pan. Simmer to halve the juice, until it is syrupy and has a strong taste.

Add the stock and tomato purée to the steak pan and bring to a boil, then add the corn-flour paste to thicken your sauce, add it a little at a time until the desired consistency has been achieved. Attach some of the resting steak juices, and eat with the grilled carrots, broccoli, onion rings, and red wine sauce.

TO COOK TIMES STEAK

TENDERLOIN: 11/2-INCH-THICK (3.5CM)

• Blue: On each side for about 11/2 minutes

• Rare: Every side about 21/4 minutes

• Middle-rare: 31/4 minutes every hand

• Medium: Each side for about 41/2 minutes

SIRLOIN STEAK: 3/4-INCH-THICK (2CM)

• Blue: Each hand for about 1 minute

• Rare: On either hand for about 11/2 minutes

• Medium-rare: 2 minutes or so each hand

• Medium: Each side about 21/4 minutes

Kidney Bean Mole With Potato Backed

SERVICE 1

1/4 cup (40 g) red, finely chopped onion

1 Teaspoon of fresh ginger, finely chopped

2 Cloves of garlic, finely chopped

1 Thai chili, finely chopped

1 cup of extra virgin olive oil

1 Teaspoon of turmeric powder

1 Teaspoon cumin in the ground

Pinch of clove at ground

Pinch of cinnamon

1 Medium Potto baker

Cup 7/8 (190 g) canned-cut tomatoes

1 Tablespoon of brown sugar

1/3 cup (50 g) red bell pepper, cored, trimmed seeds and chopped roughly

Vegetable stock: 5/8 cup (150ml)

1 Table litre of cocoa powder

1 Sesame seeds in tablespoon

2 Teaspoons of peanut butter (smooth if available, but strong chunky)

7/8 cup (150 g) of frozen reindeer

2 Tablespoons (5 g) of chopped parsley

Heat up the oven to 200oC (400 ° F).

In a medium saucepan, fry the onion, ginger , garlic and chili in the oil over medium heat for about 10 minutes, or until soft. Remove the seasoning and finish cooking for another 1 to 2 minutes.

Place the potato on a baking tray in the hot oven and bake until soft in the middle (or longer depending on how crispy you like the outside) for 45 to 60 minutes.

In the meantime, add to the casserole the tomatoes, sugar, red pepper, stock, cocoa powder, sesame seeds, peanut butter, and kidney beans and cook gently for 45 to 60 min.

To finish sprinkle with the parsley. Break the potato in two, then pour the mole over it.

Omelet-Sirtfood

SERVICE 1

About 2 ounces (50 g) streaky sliced bacon (or 2 rashers, smoked or regular, depending on your taste)

3 Medium-sized Eggs

11/4 ounces (35 g) red, thinly sliced endive

2 Table cubits (5 g) of parsley, finely chopped

1 Turmeric Tablespoon

1 cup of extra virgin olive oil

Heat up a frying pan with a nonstick. Cut the bacon into thin strips and cook until it is crispy over high heat. You don't need to add any oil, the bacon contains enough fat for cooking. Remove from the oven, and put any extra fat on a paper towel. Wipe clean cup.

Whisk the eggs and mix the endive, the parsley and the turmeric together. Cut the cooked bacon into cubes, and stir in the eggs.

In the frying pan, heat the oil-the pan should be hot but not smoking. Add the egg mixture, and move it around the pan using a spatula to start cooking the egg. Keep the fried egg bits going, and rotate around the pan until the omelet number is even. Reduce heat, and allow the omelet to firm. Ease the spatula around the edges and fold in half the omelet, or roll up and serve.

Baked Breast Chicken With Walnut And Parsley Pesto And Red Onion Salad

SERVICE 1

Petersil: 3/8 cup (15 g)

1/8 Cup Walnuts (15 g)

4 Parmesan cheese spoonfuls (15 g), rubbed

1 litre, extra virgin olive oil

1/2 lemon juice

3 spoonfuls (50ml) of water

51/2 ounces (150 g) skinless breast of chicken

1/8 cup (20 g) of red, finely sliced onions

1 Tablespoon of red wine,

11/4 ounces Arugula (35 g)

Cherry tomatoes, 2/3 cup (100 g), half cut

1 Balsamic vinegar in tablespoon

To make the pesto, put the parsley, walnuts, parmesan, olive oil, half the lemon juice, and a little water in a food processor or blender and mix until a smooth paste is in place. Gradually add more water until you get the consistency you prefer.

In the refrigerator, marinate the chicken breast in 1 tablespoon of pesto and the remaining lemon juice for 30 minutes, longer if possible.

Preheat to 400oF (200oC) on burner.

Heat a frying pan which is ovenproof over medium to high heat. In its marinade, fry the chicken on either side for 1 minute, then transfer the saucepan to the oven and cook for 8 minutes or until cooked.

Marinate the onions for 5 to 10 minutes in a red wine vinegar. Drain gas.

When cooked, remove the chicken from the oven, spoon another tablespoon of pesto over it, and let the chicken heat melt the pesto. Cover with foil and leave for 5 minutes to rest before serving.

Combine the balsamic vinegar with the arugula, tomatoes, and onion and drizzle. Serve with the chicken and spoon over the pesto left over.

Salad De Waldorf

85

SERVICE 1

1 cup (100 g) of celery, roughly chopped, including leaves

1/2 cup (50 g) of apple, chopped roughly

3/8 cup (50 g) walnuts, diced roughly

1 Tablespoon (10 g) of red onion, loosely chopped

2 Tablespoons (5 g) of chopped parsley

1 Tablelit capers

1 litre, extra virgin olive oil

1 Balsamic vinegar in tablespoon

1/4 Lemon Juice

1/4 Dijon Teaspoon Mustard

Around 2 ounces (50 g) of rye

About 11/2 ounces (35 g) of leaves are endive

Mix with the parsley and capers, the celery and its leaves, apple, walnuts, and onion.

To make the dressing whisk the sugar, vinegar, lemon juice and mustard in a pot.

Serve the combination of celery on top of the rug and endive with the seasoning and drizzle over.

Roasted Eggplant Wedges With Walnut And Parsley Pesto And Tomato Salad

SERVES 1

Petersil: 1/2 cup (20 g)

Walnuts: 3/4 ounces (20 g)

1/8 cup (20 g) Parmesan cheese (or use an alternative vegetarian or vegan), grated

1 litre, extra virgin olive oil

1/4 Lemon Juice

3 spoonfuls (50ml) of water

1 Medium aubergine (about 51/2 ounces or 150 g), quartered

1/8 cup (20 g) raw, sliced onion

1 Teaspoon (5ml) vinegar of red wine

11/4 ounces Arugula (35 g)

Cherry tomatoes: 2/3 cup (100 g)

1 Balsamic vinegar in teaspoon (5ml)

Oven gas to 400oF (200oC).

Place the parsley, walnuts, parmesan, olive oil and half the lemon juice in a food processor or blender to make the pesto and combine until you have a smooth paste. Gradually add the water until you have the correct consistency — it should be thick enough for the eggplant to stick to.

Brush the eggplant with some pesto, then leave the remainder to eat. Place on a baking tray and roast for 25 to 30 minutes, until the brown, soft, and moist eggplant is golden.

Meanwhile, cover with the red wine vinegar over the red onion and set aside — this will soften and sweeten the onion. Drain the vinegar and serve.

Combine the arugula, tomatoes, and rinse the onion and drizzle the salad over the balsamic vinegar. Serve with hot eggplant, spooning over the remaining pesto.

Sirtfood Live

SERVICE 1

Pure Greek yogurt (or vegan substitute, such as soy or coconut yogurt) 3/8 cup (100 g)

6 Half walnut

8 to 10 Medium Hulled Strawberries

Pinch of kale, stalks removed

3/4 ounce (20 g) dark chocolate (85% solids in cocoa)

1 Date to Medjool, pitted

1/2 cubic teaspoon of turmeric

Small sliver of Thai chilli (1 to 2 mm)

7/8 cup of unsweetened almond milk (200ml)

In a blender, blast all the ingredients until creamy.

Whole-Wheat Stuffed Pita

SERVICE 1

Whole-wheat pitas are a perfect way to bring in a fast lunch or easy and compact packed meal a lot of Sirtfoods. You can mess around and get imaginative with sizes, but basically all you do is put the ingredients in and it's ready to go.

OPTION TO A MEAT

3 ounces (80 g) slices of cooked turkey, chopped

Cheddar cheese: 3/4 ounce (20 g), diced

1/4 cup (35 g), diced cucumber

1/4 cup (35 g) red, chopped onion

1 Ounce (25 g), sliced arugula

11/2 to 2 tablespoons (10 to 15 g) of roughly chopped walnuts

TO THE DRESSION

1 litre, extra virgin olive oil

1 Pound of balsamic vinegar

Dash of orange juice

OPTION To A VEGAN

2 or 3 spoonfuls of hummus

1/4 cup (35 g), diced cucumber

1/4 cup (35 g) red, chopped onion

1 Ounce (25 g), sliced arugula

11/2 to 2 tablespoons (10 to 15 g) of roughly chopped walnuts

DRESSING TO THE VEGAN

1 litre, extra virgin olive oil

Lemon-juice sprint

Butternut Squash With Buckwheat And Date Tagine

Support 4

3 Extra virgin olive oil Teaspoons

1 Red, finely chopped onion

1 Tablespoon of new ginger, finely chopped

4 Cloves of garlic, finely chopped

2 Thai, finely chopped chilies

1 Tablespoon cumin in the ground

1 Stick of Cinnamon

2 Tablespoons of turmeric soil

2 x 14-ounce cans of chopped tomatoes (400 g each),

11/4 cups (300ml) vegetable stock

2/3 cup (100 g) Medjool seeds, pitted and chopped

1 x 14-ounce tin (400 g) of chickpeas, drained and rinsed

21/2 cups (500 g) butternut squash, peeled and sliced into bite-size pieces

11/4 cups (200 g) buckwheat

2 teaspoons (5 g) new coriander, chopped

1/4 cup (10 g) fresh, chopped parsley

Oven gas to 400oF (200oC).

Fry the onion, ginger , garlic, and chili in two teaspoons of the oil for 2 to 3 minutes. Add the cumin and cinnamon and 1 tablespoon of the turmeric, and cook for another 1 to 2 minutes.

Attach the tomatoes, stock, bananas, and chickpeas and simmer gently for 45 to 60 minutes. You can have to apply a little water from time to time to maintain a smooth, moist consistency and to make sure the pan will not run dry.

Place the squash in a roasting pan, mix with the remaining oil, and roast for 30 minutes until soft and charred around the edges.

Towards the end of the cooking time for the tagine, cook the buckwheat with the remaining tablespoon of turmeric according to the package instructions.

Add the roasted squash and coriander and parsley to the tagine, and serve with buckwheat.

Butter Bean And Miso Dip With Celery Sticks ...

SERVES 4

2 x 14-ounce cans of butter beans (400 g each), drained and rinsed

3 spoonfuls of extra virgin olive oil

2 Spoonfuls of brown miso paste

1/2 unwaxed lemon juice and 1/2 grated zest

4 Medium scallions, finely chopped and trimmed

1 Clove of garlic, crushed

1/4 Thai pepper, finely chopped

Sticks to celery, to serve

Celery sticks, to serve

Just mash the first seven ingredients and a potato masher until you have a coarse mixture.

Serve the celery sticks and oatcakes as a sauce.

Yogurt With Blended Walnuts, And Dark Chocolate

SERVICE 1

Around 125 g (11/3 cups) mixed berries

Pure Greek yogurt (or vegan substitute, such as soy or coconut yogurt) 2/3 cup (150 g)

1/4 cup (25 g), sliced walnuts

11/2 tablespoons (10 g) of dark chocolate (85% solids of cocoa), rinded

Only add your choice berries to a mug, then finish with the yogurt.

Sprinkle with the caramel and the walnuts.

Chicken And Broccoli Curry With Potatoes Bombay

Support 4

4 x 41/2- to 51/2-ounce (120-150 g) skinless chicken breasts, cut into pieces of bite size

4 Spoonfuls of extra virgin olive oil

3 Tablespoons of turmeric soil

2 Red, sliced onions

2 Thai, finely chopped chilies

Three cloves of garlic, finely chopped

1 Tablespoon of new ginger, finely chopped

1 Table litre of mild curry powder

Chopped tomatoes 1 x 14-ounce (400 g)

Chicken stock: 21/8 cups (500ml)

7/8 cup coconut milk (200ml)

2 Tops of cardamom

1 Stick of Cinnamon

11/3 Lbs (600 g) of russet potatoes

1/4 cup (10 g) chopped parsley

22/3 cups (175 g), sliced kale

2 Tablespoons (5 g) of chopped coriander

Rub the pieces of chicken in 1 teaspoon of oil, and 1 tablespoon of turmeric. Hang on for 30 minutes to marinate.

Fry the chicken over high heat (the chicken should be fried with ample oil in the marinade) for 4 to 5 minutes until well browned all over and fried through, then remove from the pan and set aside.

Heat 1 spoonful of the oil over medium heat in the frying pan and add the onion, chili, garlic and ginger. Fry for about 10 minutes or until tender, then add the curry powder and another turmeric tablespoon and cook for 1 to 2 minutes. Add the tomatoes to the pan and allow to cook for another 2 minutes. Remove the stock, coconut milk, cardamom and cinnamon stick and leave for 45 to 60 minutes to simmer. Check the pan frequently to ensure it doesn't run dry — you may need to add more storage.

Heat the frying pan to 425 ° F (220 ° C). Peel the potatoes while your curry is cooking, and cut them into small chunks. Place the remaining tablespoon of turmeric in boiling water, and boil for 5 minutes. Drain well, and prepare for 10 minutes of dry steam. Round the edges they should be white and flaky. Transfer to a roasting pan, stir in the remaining oil and roast until golden brown and crisp for 30 minutes. When they are ready, throw the parsley through.

Add the kale, cooked chicken, and coriander when the curry has your required consistency, and cook for another 5 minutes to ensure the chicken is cooked through, then serve with the potatoes.

Spiced Scrambled Eggs

SERVES 1

1 cup of extra virgin olive oil

1/8 cup (20 g) red, finely chopped onion

1/2 Thai pepper, finely chopped

3 Medium-sized Eggs

1/4 cup milk (50ml)

1 Teaspoon of turmeric powder

2 Table cubits (5 g) of parsley, finely chopped

In a frying pan, heat the oil and fry the red onion and chili until soft but not brown.

Whisk the eggs, the milk, the turmeric and the parsley together. Add to the hot pan and continue to cook over low to medium heat, moving the egg mixture around the pan constantly to scramble it and stop it from sticking / burning. Serve when you have achieved the consistency you desire.

Chili Con Carne Sirt

Support 4

1 Red, finely chopped onion

Three cloves of garlic, finely chopped

2 Thai, finely chopped chilies

1 litre, extra virgin olive oil

1 Tablespoon cumin in the ground

1 Tablespoon of turmeric soil

Lean beef (5 per cent fat) 1 pound (450 g)

Red wine: 5/8 cup (150ml)

1 Red bell potato, cored, seeds removed and cut into bits of bite size

Chopped tomatoes 2 x 14-ounce (400 g) cans

1 Tomato cubit purée

1 Table litre of cocoa powder

7/8 cup (150 g) of frozen reindeer

Beef stock: 11/4 cups (300ml)

2 Tablespoons (5 g) fresh, chopped coriander

2 Tablespoons (5 g) of fresh, chopped parsley

1 Cup Buckwheat (160 g)

Fry the onion, garlic, and chili in the oil for 2 to 3 minutes over medium heat in a large saucepan, then add the spices and cook for another minute or two. Add the ground beef and cook over medium-high heat for 2 to 3 minutes until the meat is well browned throughout. Add the red wine, and allow it to bubble to halve it.

Add the red pepper, tomatoes, purée tomatoes, cocoa, kidney beans and stock and leave for 1 hour to simmer. Occasionally, you would need to apply a little water to maintain a dense, sticky consistency. Stir in the chopped herbs, just before serving.

Meanwhile, according to the package instructions, cook the buckwheat and serve alongside the chilli.

Scramble Mushroom And Tofu

SERVICE 1

31/2 ounces (100 g) of tofu extra firm

1 Teaspoon of turmeric powder

1 cup of mild curry powder

1/3 cup (20 g) kale, chopped roughly

1 cup of extra virgin olive oil

1/8 cup (20 g) red, thinly sliced onion

1/2 Thai Chili, with thin slices

Mushrooms: 3/4 cup (50 g), thinly sliced

2 Table cubits (5 g) of parsley, finely chopped

Wrap the tofu in paper towels and top with something heavy to help drain it.

Mix the curry and turmeric powder, then add a little water until a light paste has been achieved. Steam the Kale for two or three minutes.

Heat the oil over medium heat in a frying pan and fry the onion, chili and mushrooms for 2 to 3 minutes until browning and softening has begun.

Crumble the tofu into pieces of bite size and add to the saucepan, pour over the tofu the spice mix and thoroughly mix. Cook for 2 to 3 minutes over medium heat so that the spices are cooked through and the tofu has begun browning. Add the kale, and continue cooking for another minute over medium heat. Add the parsley, mix well and serve.

Salmon Pasta Smoked With Chili And Arugula

Support 4

2 Spoonfuls of extra virgin olive oil

1 Red, finely chopped onion

2 Cloves of garlic, finely chopped

2 Thai, finely chopped chilies

1 cup (150 g) of cherry tomatoes, cut in half

1/2 cup white wine (100ml)

Buckwheat pasta: 9 to 11 ounces (250 to 300 g)

9 Ounces Smoked Salmon (250 g)

2 Capers spoons

1⁄2 lemon juice

2 Ounces Arugula (60 g)

1/4 cup (10 g) chopped parsley

In a frying pan flame 1 tablespoon of the oil over low heat. Stir in the onion, garlic, chili and fry until soft but not brown.

Add the tomatoes and allow to cook for one or two minutes. To that by half add the white wine and bubble.

Cook the pasta in boiling water with 1 tablespoon of oil for 8 to 10 minutes depending on whether you like it al dente, then rinse.

Slice the salmon into strips and add the capers, lemon juice, arugula and parsley to the tomato saucepan. Add the pasta, mix well and serve straight away. Drizzle any oil left over top.

Salad Bukkwheat Pasta

SERVICE 1

2 ounces (50 g) of buckwheat pasta, cooked according to the instructions for packaging

Large pound of rye

Tiny pound of basil leaves

8 Halved cherry tomatoes

Avocado 1/2, diked

10 Tiny olives

1 litre, extra virgin olive oil

21/2 lbs (20 g) of pine nuts

Combine all the ingredients, except the pine nuts, gently and arrange them on a plate, then scatter the nuts over the top.

Pancakes Buckwheat With Cream, Deep Chocolate Syrup, And Crushed Walnuts

Allows 6 TO 8 PANCAKES, Build ON THE Scale

For The PANCAKES

11/2 cups of milk (350ml),

Buckwheat flour: 7/8 cup (150 g)

1 Big Egg

1 spoonful of extra virgin olive oil, to cook BY THE SAUCE CHOCOLAT E

31⁄2 ounces (100 g) dark chocolate (85% solid cocoa)

1/3 cup milk (85ml)

1 Double cream c.l.

103

1 litre, extra virgin olive oil

UPDATE

2 Cups (400 g) of strawberries, diced and hulled

7/8 cup (100 g), sliced walnuts

Place all the ingredients apart from the olive oil in a blender to make the pancake batter, and combine until you have a smooth batter. It should not be too thick or excessively runny. (Any excess batter can be stored in an airtight container in your fridge for up to 5 days. Be sure to mix well before using it again.)

Melt the chocolate in a heat-proof bowl over a pan of simmering water to make the chocolate sauce. When warmed, blend well in the milk and whisk thoroughly, then apply the double cream and olive oil. By leaving the water in the pan, you can keep the sauce warm, simmering at very low heat until your pancakes are ready.

Heat a small or medium heavy-bottomed frying pan to make the pancakes, until it begins to smoke, then add the olive oil.

Place some of the batter into the middle of the tub, then tip the excess batter around it until you've coated the whole surface; you might need to add a little more batter to do that. If your pan is hot enough, you will just need to cook the pancake on either side for 1 minute or so.

Using a spatula to remove the pancake around the bottom, until you can see it go brown around the top, then turn it over. Seek to turn over to avoid splitting it in one movement. On the other hand, cook for another minute or two, and move to a tray.

Place some strawberries in the middle and turn the pancake upwards. Continue until you've made as many pancakes as possible.

Over each pancake, spoon a decent amount of sauce and scatter with some sliced walnuts.

You can find your first attempts to be too fat or to fall apart, but if you find the formula for your batter that fits better for you and you refine your technique, you'll make it like a professional. In this scenario preparation makes good.

Tofu And Shiitake Soup Mushroom

SERVES 4

1/3 ounce (10 g) dry (seaweed) wakame

1 fifth vegetable stock (1 litre)

7 Ounces (200 g) shiitake, sliced mushrooms

1/3 Cup Miso Paste (120 g)

1 x 14-ounce (400 g) firm tofu block, cut in small cubes

2 Scallions, diagonally trimmed and slipped

1 Thai, finely chopped chili (optional)

Soak the wakame 10 minutes in warm water then drain.

Bring the stock to a boil, then add the mushrooms and gently simmer for 1-2 minutes.

Dissolve the miso paste with some of the warm stock in a bowl to ensure it thoroughly dissolves. Add the miso and tofu to the remaining stock, be careful not to let the soup boil because that will spoil the delicate taste of miso. If using and serving, add the drained wakame, scallions, and chili.

Sirtfood Pizza

MAKES TWO 12-INCH, PIZZAS (30CM)

BY Pie CRUST

1 x 1/4-ounce (7 g) dry leaven packet

1 Tablespoon of brown sugar

11/4 cups of lukewarm water (300ml)

Buckwheat flour: 11/4 cups (200 g)

12/3 cups (200 g) of white bread flour or pasta flour type Tipo 00 plus a little extra to spread out

1 spoonful of extra virgin olive oil, plus a little extra to grease

OF THE SAUCE TOMATO

1/2 red, finely chopped onion

1 Clove of garlic, finely chopped

1 cup of extra virgin olive oil

1 Liter of dried oregano

2 Cups of white wine

Pot of sliced tomatoes 1 x 14-ounce (400 g)

Pinch of brunette sugar

2 Spoonfuls (5 g) of basil leaves

YOUR TOPPING FAVORITE

• Red onion, arugula, grated cheese (or vegan alternatives), and grilled eggplant. (You may be able to buy grilled eggplant from a local deli or market. To grill your own, heat the griddle pan until it starts to smoke, then reduce the heat to medium. Slice the eggplant crossways into thin slices no wider than 1/4 inch [3 to 5 mm], brush with a little extra virgin olive oil and cook until black grill marks are obtained on either side of the eggplant and it is nice and soft.

• Chili flakes, cherry tomatoes, goat cheese and arugula.

• Cooked chicken, rye, red onion, olive and rind cheese

• Chorizo, red onion, steamed kale and rubbed cheese

Dissolve yeast and sugar in water for the bread. This will help the yeast to become active. Cover with plastic wrap and leave ten to fifteen minutes.

Sew the flours in a pot. Complete it with the dough hook if you have a stand mixer, and sift the flours into the mixer pot.

Add the yeast mixture and oil to the flour, and combine until a dough has been formed. If your dough is a little dry you might need to add a little more water. Knead until a soft, springy dough is covered.

Shift the dough to an oiled tub, cover it with a cool , wet kitchen towel, and keep it warm somewhere to rise for 45 to 60 minutes before it is doubled.

Meanwhile, make the sauce with tomatoes. Fry the olive oil with the onion and garlic until soft, then add the dried oregano. Use the alcohol and bubble to halve.

Add the tomatoes and sugar, put back to a boil and simmer for 30 minutes until a thick consistency is achieved. If it's too runny the crust can get soggy. Delete the heat from oven. With your hands, rip the basil leaves apart and stir them into the sauce.

Start kneading the dough to expel the air again — this is called knocking out, or punching hard. If you have a nice smooth dough after a minute or so it's ready. You can either directly use the flour, or wrap it in plastic wrap and place it in the refrigerator for a few days.

Pump up the oven to 230oC (450oF). Lightly buff a floured work surface. Cut the dough in half and roll out each piece to the required thickness, then place it on a pizza stone or oiled baking tray with nonstick. (This amount of dough should produce two thin-crust pizzas about 12 inches [30 cm] in diameter. If you want a thicker crust just use some of the dough or decrease the pizza size.)

Spread a thin layer of tomato sauce over the dough (for that quantity of dough you will only need about half the sauce, but freeze any left over), leaving a gap for the crust around the edge. Add the remaining ingredients (if you use arugula and chili flakes, add them after you have baked the pizza). Until baking, set aside for around 15 to 20 minutes; the dough will begin to rise again, giving it a lighter foundation.

Bake 10 to 12 minutes in the oven, or until the cheese is golden brown. Now, if using, top it with arugula and chili flakes.

Sirtfood Bite

MAKES 15 TO BITES 20

1 Cup Walnuts (120 g)

1 ounce (30 g) of dark chocolate (85% solid cocoa), split in pieces; or 1/4 cup cocoa nibs

9 Ounces (250 g) Dates in Medjool, pitted

1 Table litre of chocolate powder

1 Tablespoon of turmeric soil

1 litre, extra virgin olive oil

1 Vanille pod or 1 teaspoon vanilla extract scraped seeds

1 or 2 spoonfuls of water

Place the walnuts and chocolate in a food processor and process them until the powder is fine.

Add all the remaining ingredients except water and combine until the mixture forms a disk. Depending on the consistency of the paste, you may or may not have to apply the water-you don't want it to be so wet.

Form the mixture into bite-size balls using your hands and cool in an airtight container for at least 1 hour before eating them. In some more cocoa or dried coconut you could roll some of the balls to achieve a different finish, if you like. They will keep it in your fridge for up to 1 week.

Part 2

What Is Sirtfood And Sirtuin Anyway?

Before we even get to the diet, let's discuss the main ingredients of the sirtfood diet. The part of the name Sirt is no accident, because it is derived from the enzyme sirtuin. Sirtuin is a natural enzyme, or a natural protein, which has a positive effect on our body. For example, it is responsible for protecting the cells from dying quickly. But the protection against inflammation also falls within the scope of the sirtuin.

Sirtuin is still largely unknown among the general population, but science has already put out feelers here and there. It was found out that sirtuin can have a targeted effect on the metabolism. With this enzyme it is quite possible that you speed up your metabolism. In addition, the muscle mass, more precisely the effectiveness of the individual muscle fibers, is increased by the protein sirtuin. Some even speak of a makeover, and that's not really surprising. Finally, sirtuin also works against cell damage. Quite simply, it can be summarized that the sirtuin has a very positive effect on the human body.

But where does the sirtuin actually come from? It comes from herbal products and is no coincidence either. Sirtuin is released by plants that are stressed. This is the case when the environmental conditions change or when someone moves on to the greenery. Now you can surely imagine that the plant is very stressed if we simply cut off a few vegetables or, for example, pull a carrot out of the ground, i.e. take away its natural plant environment. The carrot in this case reacts with stress and pours out sirtuin. However, since we plan to eat this carrot, we logically include the sirtuin and that is exactly what it is about.

So What's Up With Sirtuin?

Sirtuin is vital for the human body because we use the enzyme when we are stressed ourselves. In addition, sirtuinhelps not only maintain weight but also it decrease. Even the brain needs sirtuin in order to be able to fully utilize its storage capacity. After all, the protein protects the neurons and thus provides good protection against certain diseases, such as Alzheimer's.

However, the latest research also shows that sirtuin can protect against diabetes. The more sirtuin diabetics ingest, the greater the protective effect of the protein.

I already told you that sirtuin can also be seen as a fountain of youth. For example, Sirtuin protects against cell breakdown and healthy and protected cells mean smooth, radiant skin! Sirtuin is a very special enzyme and it is actually no wonder that there is increasing interest in how it works. This is what happened to the two researchers Aidan Goggins and Glen Metten, who also launched the sirtfood diet on the side. The two scientists really only wanted to find out more about this enzyme. It is good for us who want to lose weight that they founded the sirtfood diet.

This Is How The Sirtfood Diet Works

You already know what the sirtuin is all about. The enzyme has a positive effect on the body and this is exactly what the sirtfood diet uses for itself. As you already know, sirtuin is a protein and here we are slowly approaching the low-carb diet, because it is also based on proteins. However, the sirtfood diet does not excludeautomatically products such as bread. Rather, it depends on the products that contain a lot of sirtuin.

And that is exactly the essence of the sirtfood diet. Mainly sirtuin-containing foods should be eaten, as these have a positive effect on the metabolism and on weight. According to the two scientists Aidan Goggins and Glen Metten, up to 3 kilograms per week should melt after the sirtfood diet. However, the diet is divided into 3 phases. I would like to describe these three phases to you in more detail so that you understand the principle of the sirtfood diet.

Phase 1

The first phase lasts 3 days. In this phase, you are allowed to consume 1000 kilocalories a day. You shouldn't consume these carelessly, but with sirtuin-containing juices and smoothies, as well as a main meal a day. A small snack is also provided, but only if the 1000 kilocalories are not exceeded.

Day 1				
In the morning	Noon	in the evening	snack	Additionally
Smoothie e.g. celery smoothie (105 kcal)	Spicy salmon (480 kcal)	Smoothie, for example Orange pineapple smoothie (132 kcal)	Menti snack (119 kcal)	1 smoothie E.g. fruit cocktail smoothie (132 kcal)
Day 2				
In the morning	Noon	in the evening	snack	Additionally
Smoothie e.g. orange smoothie	Tropical vegetable salad (360 kcal)	Smoothie e.g. kiwi smoothie (363 kcal)	KiLiGra	-

116

(142 kcal)			(213 kcal)	
Day 3				
In the morning	Noon	in the evening	snack	Additionally
Smoothie E.g. blue coconut smoothie (186 kcal)	Pesto lunch (464 kcal)	**Smoothie e.g. turmeric smoothie (76 kcal)**	Chili Lemon Olives (110 kcal)	1 smoothie e.g. Red raspberry smoothie (176 kcal)

When you have read in, you can also deal with the nutrition plan in more detail and put together your personal nutrition plan, the way it tastes to you and you feel comfortable with it. In the first phase, it is only important that you stick to the 1000 calories!

Phase 2

The second phase is not dissimilar to the first phase. However, there are some differences here. In addition to the fact that you can now have two main meals in this phase, you shouldalso increase your daily calorie requirement to 1500 kcal per day but the sirtuin-containing smoothies and juices play an important role. All the calories that you haven't used up with the recipes for lunch and dinner can be filled with smoothies and juices. Incidentally, the duration of the second phase is quite controversial. Some claim that the second phase lasts until you reach your desired weight. This is very individual and therefore, it is not surprising that an individual period of time for the second phase inevitably occurs but let's assume that you want to lose 3 kilos, then the second phase lasts from day 4 to day 7. Your nutrition plan could look like this:

Day 4				
In the morning	Noon	in the evening	snack	Additionally
Strawberry smoothie (85 kcal)	Sirt steak salad (441 Kcal)	**Winter vegetable soup (289 kcal)**	Solid red (65 kcal)	Smoothies around 1500 kcal
Day 5				
In the morning	Noon	in the evening	snack	Additionally

Fresh, sweet and sour smoothie (38 kcal)	Baked sweet potato with feta, radishes and cress (563 kcal)	**Neptune salad** **(379 kcal)**	Sirt-Snack-Deluxe (141 kcal)	Smoothies around 1500 kcal

Day 6

In the morning	Noon	**in the evening**	snack	Additionally
Pink buttermilk smoothie (65)	Quinoa lunch with chicken (592 kcal)	**Hohenzollern pan** **(239 kcal)**	Green toasted snack (255 kcal)	Smoothies around 1500 kcal

Day 7

In the morning	Noon	**in the evening**	snack	Additionally
Green surprise smoothie (363 kcal)	Tropical vegetable salad	**Stew with green vegetables**	Celery sticks with	Smoothies around 1500 kcal

	(360 kcal)	**(380 kcal)**	yogurt dip (97 kcal)	

Phase 3

The third phase is very similar to the second phase. However, the third phase is less of a model and more of a permanent change in diet. This is used to avoid the yo-yo effect. In the third phase, you can draw on the full, so there are 3 meals a day and smoothies or juices that do not exceed 1800 kcal per day. You can continue this phase for several days and then gradually taper off the sirtfood diet. But you can just as easily continue it permanently. So that you understand how this is meant in detail, I would like to show you a day in the sirtfood diet in the third phase:

Day 8 and following				
In the morning	Noon	in the evening	snack	Additionally
Chia coconut pudding with chia and	Salad a la sirtuinfood (304 kcal)	Far Eastern curry (488	Kale chips with peanuts	Smoothies to reach 1800 kcal

120

blueberri es (297 kcal)		kcal)	(160 kcal)	

You can let your imagination run wild and combine yourself to your 1800 kcal per day. There are no limits to your creativity. You can also use the recipes from the book in a variety of ways.

Sirtuin-Rich Foods And Where To Find Them

Not everyone likes everything and most diets have one major drawback: they consist mainly of what you don't like and categorically exclude all other goodies! It's good that the sirtfood diet works a little differently. You have a large selection of different foods that you can and should eat. In fact, chocolate also counts here, as you can see in the table.

So the sirtfood diet is very versatile and varied and that makes it a special diet. The good thing about it: You can also swap the ingredients for one another. For example, if you don't particularly like blueberries or blueberries, then choose raspberries instead. Until you get a feel for it, you should stick to the recipes in this book. There will still be enough leeway for your own creations.

So what are all the foods that contain high levels of the enzyme sirtuin? You can easily take this from the table.

Fruit	<ul><li>Blueberries</li><li>Strawberries</li><li>Raspberries</li><li>Apples</li><li>Citrus fruits</li><li>Blue plums</li><li>Blue grapes</li><li>Blackberries</li><li>Goji berries</li><li>Kumquats</li><li>Black currants</li></ul>
Vegetables	<ul><li>broccoli</li><li>celery</li><li>Red onions</li><li>arugula</li><li>Kale</li><li>Chilies</li><li>Chicory</li><li>artichokes</li><li>Watercress</li><li>endive salad</li><li>Pak choi</li><li>Green beans</li><li>asparagus</li><li>Shallots</li></ul>

	• Field beans • White beans
Spices	• garlic • chili • ginger • Turmeric, • cinnamon • curry
Beverages	• Green tea • coffee • red wine • water • Black tea • White teas
Cereals, nuts and seeds	• Buckwheat • Walnuts • Popcorn • Quinoa • Whole wheat flour • Chia seeds • peanuts • Sweet chestnuts • Pecans • Pistachios • Sunflower seeds
Herbs	• parsley • oregano • basil • thyme

	• rosemary • dill • sage • peppermint • chives
Goodies	• Dark chocolate, min. 85% cocoa content • Olives • Capers • Dates • native olive oil

A large selection! So you can reach your desired weight with no regrets and with pleasure. What is about hunger?

Lose Weight Without Hunger

The sirt food diet is a special form of low-carb diet. If you have already dealt with different diets then you also know about low carb. For example, the low-carb diet is also based on proteins. The enzyme sirtuin is not specifically emphasized here. However, sirtuin is also a protein and what else do proteins have in them? Exactly! They fill us up. But it is not an unpleasant feeling of satiety, but a feeling of well-being and that even lasts. Unlike eating white bread for breakfast, the body takes much longer to process protein. Simple carbohydrates like those found in white bread are far too easily accessible for the body. Incidentally, this also leads to the fact that the blood sugar level rises and falls quickly and you get hungry again very quickly or even suffer a ravenous hunger attack! If you stick to the rules of the game, both are almost impossible with the sirtfood diet!

So it is quite possible that you are completely full, feel good and do not have to go hungry and still lose weight!

A Few Tips Before You Start

Whether we are talking about a change in diet, it does not matter at first - it is a change in known habits either way. Because of this, many people find it difficult to persevere and pull off a change in diet. This does not only apply to the sirtfood diet, it is universal. So that you can master the start of the sirtfood diet more easily, it is recommended that you reduce your daily calories about 2 weeks before the planned start of the sirtfood diet and not suddenly, but bit by bit. For 2 or 3 days, watch yourself how many calories you eat each day. Assume you consume 2200 kcal per day. Of the 14 days, there are now 11 days left to reduce your daily calories. According to this simple calculation, you have to save almost 190 kcal every day. In this way, you gently get to the 1,000 kcal allowed in the first phase and do not have to make a brutal start. Incidentally, this also promotes stamina enormously and your body is not pushed into cold water and does not even know what is happening to it.

If you'd rather have more time to prepare, you can start much earlier, observe yourself longer and reduce your calorie intake even more slowly. Here you and your personal preference are asked! You can then gradually begin to eliminate empty carbohydrates, such as sugar or white flour, from your diet. This will also make it easier for you in the future and you will soon notice how different life can taste!

But enough of the long speech. Surely you are curious about all the recipes and that's why the delicious recipes from this book are now following!

The Recipes

Here I would like to finally introduce you to the recipes that will make your sirtfood diet a pleasure. In spite of the fact that one would think that the sirtfood diet offers little variety, it is very astonishing what variation and diversity there is in the sirtfood diet.

The recipes are structured in such a way that you are not tied to the nutrition plan already shown, but that you can put together your own nutrition plan yourself. Please always pay attention to the phase you are in so that you do not exceed the permitted calorie intake. Otherwise the sirtfood diet will not bring the desired results.

So you will find recipes in this section for the following points:

- Smoothies
- Breakfast
- Having lunch
- Dinner and
- Snacks

Try the recipes and get to know a whole new way of life: finally weight loss with pleasure and without sacrificing!

I wish you will be the best of luck with cooking the recipes and a special culinary highlight - every day anew!

Smoothies

Orange Smoothie

Preparation time 5 minutes

Difficulty very easy

Servings 2 servings

Per serving

Calories 142 kcal

Protein 18 g

Fat 2 g

Carbohydrates 9 g

Ingredients

2 oranges

1 small grapefruit

200 ml carrot juice

80 g low-fat quark (4 tbsp)

1 teaspoon rapeseed oil

Preparation

Squeeze oranges and grapefruit vigorously (should make about 200 ml and 100 ml).

Pour orange and grapefruit juice with carrot juice, low-fat quark and oil into a tall mixing vessel and puree until smooth with a hand blender. Drink cold immediately.

Blue Coconut Smoothie

Preparation time 10 minutes

Difficulty very easy

Servings 2 servings

Per serving

Calories 186 kcal

Protein 23 g

Fat 5 g

Carbohydrates 3 g

Ingredients

1 banana

2 dried dates (pitted)

1 teaspoon coconut oil

150 g blueberries

300 ml almond drink (almond milk)

1 pinch of cinnamon

2 teaspoons coconut flakes

3 fresh mint leaves

Preparation

Remove the peel from the banana and cut into pieces. Split the dates into two and remove the core.

Pour coconut oil together with banana, dates, blueberries, almond milk, cinnamon and desiccated coconut into a suitable container and puree everything at the highest level until the smoothie takes on the desired consistency.

Pour blue coconut smoothie into 2 glasses and enjoy garnished with desiccated coconut and mint.

Pomegranate And Cranberry Smoothie

Preparation time 10 minutes

Difficulty very easy

Servings 2 servings

Per serving

Calories 152 kcal

Protein 17 g

Fat 4 g

Carbohydrates 9 g

Ingredients

1 pomegranate

100 g cranberries

150 g yogurt (1.5% fat)

Liquid sweetener at will

250 ml milk (1.5% fat)

Ice cubes

Preparation

Cut a wedge-shaped piece from the stalk of the pomegranate. Then breakcarefully the fruit into two parts over a bowl with a little pressure so that most of the stones fall out of the shell. If necessary, work the pomegranate with thin rubber or disposable gloves, as the juice is very colored.

Set aside about 1 tbsp of the pomegranate seeds. Pour the rest with the cranberries and yoghurt into a suitable mixing vessel and puree with a hand blender. Add a little sweetener to your own taste, stir in the milk and ice cubes and mix in again briefly with the hand blender. Divide between 2 glasses and serve garnished with the remaining pomegranate seeds.

Orange Pineapple Smoothie

Preparation time 10 minutes

Difficulty very easy

Servings 2 servings

Per serving

Calories 132 kcal

Protein 16 g

Fat 0 g

Carbohydrates 7 g

Ingredients

200 g yoghurt, natural 3.8%

50 g pineapple raw

40 g of orange

50 g banana

50 ml drinking water as required

1 teaspoon lemon juice (freshly squeezed)

1 teaspoon agave syrup as required

Preparation

Separate the peel of the pineapple generously and remove the hard center piece from the pineapple, then divide into pieces. Remove the orange from the peel. Remove the peel of the banana and roughly cut or break into pieces.

Pour the pineapple, orange and banana with yoghurt and water into a suitable mixing vessel and puree. Sweeten the fruit smoothie with lemon and agave syrup according to your own preference and divide it into two glasses.

Turmeric Smoothie

Preparation time 5 minutes

Difficulty very easy

Servings: 1 serving

Per serving

Calories 76 kcal

Protein 16 g

Fat 0 g

Carbohydrates 1 g

Ingredients

200 g papaya

2 tbsp fresh lime juice

1 teaspoon turmeric powder

200 ml tap water

Preparation

Cut the papaya in half and remove the seeds from the inside with a spoon. Take the pulp of the papaya out of the skin and fill it into a suitable mixing vessel. Add lime juice, turmeric and water to the mixing vessel and puree everything until smooth. Pour the papaya smoothie into a glass and enjoy immediately.

Green Banana Smoothie

Preparation time 10 minutes

Difficulty very easy

Servings 1 serving

Per serving

Calories 261 kcal

Protein 23 g

Fat 14 g

Carbohydrates 8 g

Ingredients

60 g fresh avocado Hass

30 g fresh baby spinach

70 g banana

2 dates

100 ml drinking water as required

Preparation

Cut the avocado in two and remove the core from the pulp, then spoon the pulp out of the skin and pour into a suitable mixing vessel. Rinse the spinach leaves. Remove the peel from the banana and break it into large pieces.

Add the spinach, banana and pitted dates to the avocado in the mixing vessel. Puree everything with the hand blender, adding a little more water if necessary until the desired consistency is achieved. Pour the green smoothie into a glass and enjoy immediately.

Red Raspberry Smoothie

Preparation time 5 minutes

Difficulty very easy

Servings 2 servings

Per serving

Calories 176 kcal

Protein 18 g

Fat 9 g

Carbohydrates 4 g

Ingredients

125 g raspberries

50 g yoghurt, natural 1.8%

25 g ground almonds

25 g oatmeal

1 stalk of mint

100 ml organic soy drink

200 ml drinking water as required

Preparation

Rinse the raspberries and let them dry. Wash off the mint and strip the leaves from the stem. Put aside 4 leaves for the garnish. Put the remaining mint leaves with the raspberries, yoghurt, almonds and oat flakes in a suitable mixing vessel.

Add milk or nut drink and 100 ml water and puree everything until smooth. If the smoothie is still too thick, just add some more water and mix it again with the hand blender. Pour the raspberry smoothie into two glasses and serve with a little oat flakes and mint leaves.

Celery Smoothie

Preparation time 10 minutes

Difficulty very easy

Servings 1 serving

Per serving

Calories 105 kcal

Protein 3 g

Fat 0 g

Carbohydrates 20 g

Ingredients

1 stick of celery (celery), raw

1 apple

50 g fresh baby spinach

1 dates

200 ml drinking water as required

Preparation

Wash the celery stalk, apple and baby spinach and let drain. Clean the celery stalk again and cut into large pieces. Cut the apple in half, remove the core from the apple and cut into large pieces.

Put the celery, apple, spinach and the date in a suitable mixing vessel, fill up with 200 ml water and puree until smooth. Pour the smoothie into a glass and serve.

Kiwi Smoothie

Preparation time 5 minutes

Difficulty very easy

Servings 1 serving

Per serving

Calories 363 kcal

Protein 15 g

Fat 28 g

Carbohydrates 9 g

Ingredients

1 kiwi

10 g cashew nuts

30 g spinach

½ avocado

½ apple

1 stalk of mint

1 splash of freshly squeezed lime juice

200 ml of water

Preparation

Wash off the spinach, apple and mint and leave to dry. Cut out the core of the apple and cut the apple into pieces. Remove the pulp of the avocado from the skin and dice. Divide the kiwi lengthways and use a spoon to remove the pulp from the skin.

Pour the kiwi, spinach, apple, avocado, mint, lime juice and cashew nuts with 200 ml of water into a suitable mixing vessel and puree finely with the hand blender. Pour the smoothie into a glass and serve.

Tropical Smoothie

Preparation time 10 minutes

Difficulty very easy

Servings 2 servings

Per serving

Calories 189 kcal

Protein 4 g

Fat 18 g

Carbohydrates 4 g

Ingredients

1 fresh avocado

100 g honeydew melon

2 tbsp coconut oil

2 stalks of mint

100 ml tap water as needed

Preparation

Halve the avocado lengthways and remove the pulp from the skin with a spoon. Separate the melon from the skin and pour into a suitable mixing vessel together with the avocado and coconut oil.

Wash off the mint, pat dry and add to the mixing bowl. Puree everything well, add a little water if necessary and serve in a glass.

Strawberry Smoothie

Preparation time 10 minutes

Difficulty very easy

Servings 2 servings

Per serving

Calories 85 kcal

Protein 7 g

Fat 12 g

Carbohydrates 1 g

Ingredients

150 g strawberries

25 g whey protein powder vanilla

100 g soy yogurt

200 ml of drinking water

Preparation

Clean and trim the strawberries and remove the base of the calyx. Put all ingredients in a tall mixing vessel and puree until smooth. Pour the smoothie into two glasses and enjoy chilled

Fruit Cocktail Smoothie

Preparation time 10 minutes

Difficulty very easy

Servings 2 servings

Per serving

Calories 132 kcal

Protein 17 g

Fat 6 g

Carbohydrates 0 g

Ingredients

200 g yoghurt, natural 3.8%

50 g pineapple raw

40 g of orange

50 g banana

50 ml drinking water as required

1 teaspoon lemon juice (freshly squeezed)

1 teaspoon agave syrup as required

Preparation

Remove the peel from the pineapple and cut out the hard center piece, then cut into pieces. Peel off the peel of the orange. Remove the banana from the peel and roughly cut into pieces.

Put the pineapple, orange and banana with yoghurt and water in a tall mixing vessel and puree until smooth. Sweeten the fruit smoothie with lemon and agave syrup as required, divide it into two glasses and enjoy immediately.

Green Surprise Smoothie

Preparation time 5 minutes

Difficulty very easy

Servings 1 serving

Per serving

Calories 363 kcal

Protein 25 g

Fat 22 g

Carbohydrates 6 g

Ingredients

1 kiwi

10 g cashew nuts

30 g spinach

½ avocado

½ apple

1 stalk of mint

1 splash of lime juice(freshly squeezed)

200 ml of water

Preparation

Clean the spinach, apple and mint and allow to dry. Remove the core of the apple and cut the apple into pieces. Spoon the pulp of the avocado out of the skin and roughly cut it. Halve the kiwi horizontally and remove the flesh from the skin with a spoon.

Pour the kiwi, spinach, apple, avocado, mint, lime juice and cashew nuts with 200 ml of water into a tall mixing vessel and puree until smooth with the hand blender. Pour the smoothie into a glass and serve.

Pink Buttermilk Smoothie

Preparation time 10 minutes

Difficulty very easy

Servings 2 servings

Per serving

Calories 65 kcal

Protein 14 g

Fat 1 g

Carbohydrates 7 g

Ingredients

200 ml buttermilk

200 ml tap water

60 g raspberries

5 ml freshly squeezed lemon

5 g grated ginger

2 teaspoons agave syrup

2 stalks of mint

Preparation

Wash off the raspberries. Put the buttermilk, raspberries, lemon juice and agave syrup in a suitable mixing vessel and mix to a pulp.

Peel the ginger with a spoon and slice it finely, then add to the raspberry puree. Pour in water and mix well. Pour into two glasses and garnish with a little fresh mint. Serve and enjoy immediately.

Fresh, Sweet And Sour Smoothie

Preparation time 15 minutes

Difficulty very easy

Servings 4 servings

Per serving

Calories 38 kcal

Protein 7 g

Fat 1 g

Carbohydrates 1 g

Ingredients

300 g strawberries

200 ml of water

100 ml orange juice (freshly squeezed)

4 tbsp yogurt, 3.8%

Ice, crushed ice

Preparation

Clean, clean and let the strawberries dry. Dice 4 - 6 strawberries and set aside. Sour the mint, shake it dry and tap it lightly against the kitchen worktop, this gives the mint its full aroma, then stiffen the leaves.

Put the strawberries, orange juice and water in a tall mixing vessel and mix everything until smooth. Divide some mint leaves together with the ice into 4 glasses and then pour the smoothie over them. Place the strawberry cubes and a few mint leaves on top of the smoothie and serve immediately.

Breakfast
Plum Yoghurt Bowl With Coconut And Cocoa Nibs

Preparation time 10 minutes

Difficulty very easy

Servings 1 serving

Per serving

Calories 435 kcal

Protein 27 g

Fat 10 g

Carbohydrates 16 g

Ingredients

200 g yoghurt, natural 1.8%

100 g blue plums

10 g cocoa nibs

10 g peanuts

20 g toasted coconut chips

Agave syrup as needed

Preparation

Wash the plums, put a few aside for the topping, divide the rest in two and remove the stones. Put the pitted plums with the yoghurt in a tall mixing vessel and puree finely with the hand blender.

Depending on the sweetness of the plums, sweeten the mixture with agave syrup, then place in a bowl. Roughly chop the peanuts and garnish with the remaining plums, cocoa nibs and coconut chips on the plum yoghurt bowl.

Muesli With Yogurt And Fruits

Preparation time 45 minutes

Difficulty very easy

Servings 2 servings

Per serving

Calories 390 kcal

Protein 14 g

Fat 9 g

Carbohydrates 10 g

Ingredients

200 g Greek yogurt,

50 g strawberries

1 medium kiwi

25 g almonds

25 g peanuts

10 g fresh walnuts

10 g sunflower seeds

10 g coconut flour

1 egg white, chicken egg

1 tspXucker Premium (Finnish xylitol)

½ teaspoon of ground bourbon vanilla

1 pinch of sea salt

preparation

Crush the nuts in the moulinette, but do not grind them. Alternatively, choproughly the nuts with a suitable knife. Put the sunflower seeds, nuts, flour, xucker, vanilla, salt and egg white in a bowl and mix well.

Sprinkle the muesli mixture on a baking sheet lined with baking paper and spread out. Roast the muesli on the middle rack in the preheated oven at 125 ° C for 20 - 30 minutes.

In between, take out the tray two or three times and stir the muesli with a spoon so that it cooks evenly until golden. Then let the muesli cool down and divide into two glasses or keep airtight until eaten.

Peel the kiwi and cut into pieces. Wash the strawberries, let them drain and cut out the stalk, then cut in two. Place the yogurt on the muesli and decorate with the fruits.

Lime Cream With Peach

Preparation time 5 minutes

Difficulty very easy

Servings 2 servings

Per serving

Calories 201 kcal

Protein 20 g

Fat 3 g

Carbohydrates 16 g

Ingredients

200 g quark (lean)

300 g yoghurt, natural 1.8%

1 fresh lime

120 g fresh yellow peach

1 teaspoon agave syrup

Preparation

Rinse and dry the lime with hot water. Use the grater to cut off the lime zest. Then cut the lime in two and squeeze out one half. Wash and drain the peaches. Then split the peaches in two, remove the core and cut into pieces.

Put the yogurt and quark in a bowl and mix. Add lime juice and zest and stir in. If required, sweeten the lime cream with agave syrup and pour into two glasses. Drape the peach pieces on the lime cream and serve.

Greek Yogurt With Chia And Blueberries

Preparation time 5 minutes

Difficulty very easy

Servings 1 serving

Per serving

Calories 297 kcal

Protein 9 g

Fat 6 g

Carbohydrates 12 g

Ingredients

150 Greek yogurt

50 g blueberries

2 tbsp chia seeds

½ tsp agave syrup(it is optional)

Preparation

Pour Greek yogurt and chia seeds into a bowl and mix together. Sweeten the yoghurt with a little agave syrup if you like.

Wash the blueberries and let them dry in the colander. Put the yogurt in a glass or bowl and drape blueberries on top.

Chia Coconut Pudding With Raspberries

Preparation time 15 minutes + 30 minutes

Difficulty very easy

Servings 2 servings

Per serving

Calories 396 kcal

Protein 11 g

Fat 17 g

Carbohydrates 11 g

Ingredients

60 g chia seeds

500 ml coconut milk (alternatively almond or soy milk)

150 g raspberries (fresh or frozen)

1 kiwi

2 - 3 stalks of fresh mint

1 teaspoon agave syrup

Preparation

Wash the raspberries and puree about 2/3 of them with the hand blender. Pour the chia seeds into the milk and mix until no more lumps can be seen. Mix the raspberry puree and agave syrup with the chia pudding and whisk well.

Let the chia pudding soak in the refrigerator for at least 30 minutes, or better overnight. Peel the kiwi and cut into pieces. Chop the mint and mix with the kiwi. Place the fruit on top of the chia pudding and garnish with mint leaves.

Plum Yogurt

Preparation time 10 minutes + 10 minutes

Difficulty very easy

Servings 2 servings

Per serving

Calories 258 kcal

Protein 8 g

Fat 10 g

Carbohydrates 32 g

Ingredients

½ lemon

200 g bananas (1 banana)

100 g blue plums

20 g walnuts (1 heaped tablespoon)

1 teaspoon sesame oil

2 teaspoons of liquid honey

300 g yogurt (1.5% fat)

½ teaspoon ground anise

Preparation

Squeeze the lemon half. Remove the banana from the peel, cut into slices and moisten with 1 teaspoon of lemon juice.

Peel and core the plums and cut the soft flesh into pieces. Chop roughly the walnuts.

In a non-stick pan let the sesame oil heat up slowly. Fry the plums and banana in it for about 1 minute over medium heat, stirring through. Then divide into 2 small bowls and let cool for 5–10 minutes.

Whisk the honey, yoghurt and aniseed together. Drizzle over the cooled fruit. Top with the chopped walnuts and serve.

Berry Bowl

Preparation time 20 minutes

Difficulty very easy

Servings 4 servings

Per serving

Calories 393 kcal

Protein 17 g

Fat 21 g

Carbohydrates 30 g

Ingredients

600 g berries (raspberries, blueberries, blackberries)

300 g small bananas (2 small bananas)

30 g acai powder (3 tbsp)

600 g yogurt alternative made from soy

200 ml almond drink (almond milk)

30 g light sesame seeds (2 tbsp)

30 g peanuts

30 g sunflower seeds (2 tbsp)

30 g pumpkin seeds (2 tbsp)

Preparation

Rinse, sort and drain the berries; Set aside 50 g each of blueberries and blackberries. Take the bananas out of the peel, break them into pieces and puree them with berries, acai powder, yoghurt alternative and almond drink to a homogeneous mass. Fill the smoothie into 4 bowls.

For draping, roast the sesame seeds with peanuts, sunflower and pumpkin seeds in a hot pan at a medium temperature. Then set aside for 3 minutes and let cool down. Drape and serve bowls with roasted seeds, nuts and kernels and the remaining blueberries and blackberries.

Quinoa For Breakfast

Preparation time 20 minutes

Difficulty very easy

Servings 2 servings

Per serving

Calories 335 kcal

Protein 14 g

Fat 9 g

Carbohydrates 48 g

Ingredients

100 g quinoa

300 ml milk or water

2 handfuls of fruit (strawberries, raspberries, blackberries)

2 tbsp peanuts

Honey to taste

Preparation

Wash the quinoa in a sieve with cold water until it runs clear.

Bring the milk to the boil and add the quinoa. Cover and simmer at low temperature for about 15 minutes until the grains are soft, stirring occasionally.

In the meantime, wash the fruit off, remove the stalk if necessary and cut it into bite-sized pieces.

Remove the quinoa from the heat, stir and let rest for another five minutes.

Divide the finished grain into two bowls, arrange the fruit and peanuts decoratively on top and drizzle with honey.

Chia Pudding With Extra Berries

Preparation time 20 minutes + 12 hours

Difficulty very easy

Servings 4 servings

Per serving

Calories 128 kcal

Protein 3 g

Fat 4 g

Carbohydrates 17 g

Ingredients

½ vanilla pod

400 ml almond drink (almond milk)

30 g chia seeds (4 tbsp)

1 pinch of ground cardamom

250 g strawberries

1 banana

1 tbsp maple syrup

Preparation

Halve the vanilla pod lengthways and scrape the vanilla pulp out of the pod with a knife. Whisk the almond drink, chia seeds, vanilla pulp and cardamom together and let rest for about 20 minutes.

Fill chia pudding into 4 glasses and cover for 12 hours, ideally overnight, place in the refrigerator to swell.

Then wash the strawberries and let them drain. Remove the banana from the skin and cut into bite-sized slices. Mix both with maple syrup and spread over the chia puddings.

Good Morning Quark

Preparation time 10 minutes

Difficulty very easy

Servings 1 serving

Per serving

Calories 235 kcal

Protein 21 g

Fat 3 g

Carbohydrates 29 g

Ingredients

150 g quark (lean)

50 g fresh or frozen strawberries

30 g blueberries

40 g of banana

1 teaspoon coconut flakes

1 tbspgoji berries

1 teaspoon flaxseed

Agave syrup as needed

Preparation

Pour the strawberries and quark into a suitable mixing vessel and puree with the hand blender to a homogeneous mass. Sweeten fruit quark according to personal taste with agave syrup or another sweetener.

Wash the blueberries and let them dry. Remove the banana from the skin and cut into bite-sized slices. Pour the strawberry quark into a bowl and decoratively drape the blueberries, banana slices, linseed, goji berries and desiccated coconut on top and serve.

Apple Porridge

Preparation time 10 minutes

Difficulty very easy

Servings 1 serving

Per serving

Calories 360 kcal

Protein 26 g

Fat 13 g

Carbohydrates 28 g

Ingredients

60 g protein porridge

1 apple

1 tbsp chia seeds

1tbsp crushed flaxseed

Preparation

Bring the water to the boil. Pour protein porridge into a bowl with a spoon and pour 120 ml of hot water over it. Stir the porridge well and let it rest for 3 - 5 minutes.

In the meantime, wash the apple, cut into four and remove the core. Finely chop the apple pieces with the grater, then stir into the porridge with the chia and flax seeds and enjoy warm.

Flakes With Peanuts And Figs

Preparation time 5 minutes

Difficulty very easy

Servings 1 serving

Per serving

Calories 564 kcal

Protein 52 g

Fat 20 g

Carbohydrates 33 g

Ingredients

1 peach

50 g raspberries

1 fig

30 g peanuts

65 g de-oiled soy flakes

250 g soy yogurt

Preparation

Put the soy flakes in a bowl. Wash the peach, fig and raspberries and let them dry. Cut the peach in half and remove the core from the pulp, then cut into slices. Cut the fig into slices.

Arrange the peach and fig slices with the raspberries on the soy flakes. Add peanuts, you can chop them if you like. Stir in the soy yogurt and mix everything together.

Tip: For a meal prep dish, mix the soy flakes with the soy yoghurt and drape the fruit cut in small pieces on top.

Blueberry Bowl

Preparation time 10 minutes

Difficulty very easy

Servings 1 serving

Per serving

Calories 545 kcal

Protein 17 g

Fat 43 g

Carbohydrates 19 g

Ingredients

250 g Greek yogurt

1 teaspoon acai powder

1 teaspoon cocoa, slightly de-oiled

40 g blueberries

1 teaspoon chia seeds

5 g desiccated coconut

1 teaspoon bee pollen

1 teaspoon walnuts

20 g coconut muesli

Agave syrup as needed

Preparation

Whisk the yogurt with acai powder and cocoa. Sweeten the yoghurt to your own taste with a little agave syrup then pour into a bowl.

Wash the blueberries and let them dry, then serve on the yogurt. Arrange chia seeds, desiccated coconut, pollen, walnuts and muesli decoratively on the bowl and serve.

Mango And Peanut Breakfast

Preparation time 15 minutes

Difficulty very easy

Servings 1 serving

Per serving

Calories 323 kcal

Protein 14 g

Fat 16 g

Carbohydrates 29 g

Ingredients

20 g whole grain oatmeal

20 g peanuts chopped

2 teaspoons agave syrup

1 pinch of cinnamon, ground

30 g mango

200 ml soy drink, organic

Preparation

Roast oatmeal and peanuts in a pan without fat, stir several times in between so that nothing burns. Pour agave syrup and cinnamon into the pan and stir in.

Spread the muesli on a large plate to cool. In the meantime, divide the mango pulp into small pieces. Pour muesli with mango and soy drink into a bowl and serve.

A Special Kind Of Breakfast Bowl

Preparation time 10 minutes

Difficulty very easy

Servings 1 serving

Per serving

Calories 261 kcal

Protein 26 g

Fat 3 g

Carbohydrates 33 g

Ingredients

200 g quark, lean

20 g frozen blueberries,

30 g raw pomegranate

1 fig

30 g of banana

5 g chia seeds

2 tbsp tap water

Preparation

Fill the berries with 2 tablespoons of tap water into a suitable mixing vessel and puree to a homogeneous mass with the hand blender. Pour the quark into a bowl and mix the berry puree into the quark.

Wash and dry the fig, then fillet it into slices. Take the banana out of the skin and cut it into bite-sized slices. Carefully knock the pomegranate seeds out of the skin.

Arrange the fig and banana slices, pomegranate seeds and the chia seeds decoratively on the berry quark and serve.

Having Lunch

A Special Lentil Soup

Preparation time 50 minutes +70 minutes

Difficulty medium

Servings 4 servings

Per serving

Calories 585 kcal

Protein 39 g

Fat 17 g

Carbohydrates 19 g

Ingredients

100 g small red onions (2 small onions)

1 clove of garlic

2 sprigs of thyme

3 tbsp olive oil

150 g red lentils

1 tbsp paprika powder (noble sweet)

1 pinch of cumin

1 tbsp tomato paste

1 l poultry stock

275 g duck breast fillet (1 duck breast fillet)

Salt pepper

200 g very small porcini mushrooms

150 ml soy cream

Preparation

Skin and chopfinely the onions and garlic. Wash off the thyme, pat dry and strip the leaves off the stem.

Put 1/2 tbsp oil in a saucepan and let it get hot. Sweat the onions and garlic in the pan until translucent. Add the lentils to the pot and sauté for 1 minute.

Sprinkle in the paprika powder and cumin. Stir in tomato paste, sweat for 30 seconds and pour the broth over it. Bring to the boil and simmer for 15 minutes at low temperature.

Slightly cut into the skin of the duck breast with a very sharp knife in a diamond shape, leaving the meat uncut. Place the breast skin side down in a pan and fry for 15 minutes at first spicy then at a low temperature.

Turn the duck breast in the pan and fry on the meat side for 2-3 minutes. Season with salt and pepper. Wrap the duck breast in aluminum foil and let it rest for 5 minutes.

Brush off the porcini mushrooms, cut off the ends of the stems if necessary, or cut large mushrooms in half. Put the rest of the oil in a pan and let it get hot. Fry the mushrooms in it, refine with salt and pepper and season with thyme.

Puree the soup until smooth using a hand blender and press a tablespoon through a not too fine sieve into a second saucepan. Stir in the soy cream into the soup, bring to the boil again and season again with salt and pepper.

Fillet the duck breast thinly into slices and serve hot with the porcini mushrooms on top of the soup.

Sirt Steak Salad

Preparation time 35 minutes

Difficulty easy

Servings 2 servings

Per serving

Calories 441 kcal

Protein 50 g

Fat 21 g

Carbohydrates 10 g

Ingredients

250 g small papaya (1 small papaya)

200 g tomatoes (3 tomatoes)

½ lemon

4 tbsp tomato juice

1 teaspoon of liquid honey

4 tbsp olive oil

5 stalks of coriander

Salt pepper

Tabasco

1 teaspoon black peppercorns

300 g rump steak (2 rump steaks)

1 teaspoon paprika powder (hot as rose)

250 g small Chinese cabbage (0.5 small Chinese cabbage)

Preparation

Remove the pulp of the papaya from the skin and scrape out the stones with a spoon. Cut the pulp into bite-sized pieces.

Wash the tomatoes, cut into four parts, cut away the stalks and remove the kernels from the tomatoes. Mix the tomatoes and papaya in a bowl.

Squeeze half a lemon. Whisk tomato juice, 1 tbsp lemon juice, honey and 2 tbsp olive oil.

Wash off the coriander, shake dry, strip the leaves from the stem, chop and stir into the tomato sauce.

Season with salt, pepper and Tabasco at your own discretion then stir into the papaya and tomato mixture.

Pound peppercorns in a mortar. Pat the steaks dry with a kitchen crepe. Season one side with paprika powder, bread both sides in ground pepper and coat lightly with salt.

Put the remaining oil in a pan and let it get hot and fry the steaks on each side at a high temperature for 3 minutes on all sides.

Remove the steaks from the pan, wrap in aluminum foil and let rest for 4 minutes.

In the meantime, wash and clean the Chinese cabbage and fillet into fine strips. Arrange on a plate and pour the papaya and tomato mixture on top. Fillet the steaks in 5 slices each and arrange draped on the salad and serve immediately.

Yellow Lentil Soup With Chili, Ginger And Turmeric

Preparation time 45 minutes

Difficulty medium

Servings 4 servings

Per serving

Calories 366 kcal

Protein 18 g

Fat 12 g

Carbohydrates 19 g

Ingredients

200 g organic yellow lentils

200 ml coconut milk

1 teaspoonred Thai curry paste

500 ml homemade vegetable stock

2 shallots

2 cloves of garlic

1 raw pepper (chili)

8 stalks of fresh coriander

2 stalks of raw white celery (celery)

10 g ginger

1 lime organic quality

1 teaspoon turmeric powder

1 tsp curry powder

1 teaspoon five spices powder

½ teaspoon cumin

1 star anise

1 teaspoon sea salt (fleur de sel)

1 pinch of black pepper

2 tbsp coconut oil

Drinking water as needed

Preparation

Peel shallots and finely dice. Skin the garlic and cut into fine slices. Wash and dry the celery and cut into thin slices.

Let the coconut oil get hot in a high pot and fry the celery in it for about 5 minutes at a medium temperature, so it will be pleasantly soft. Then add the curry paste and fry it, add the shallots and garlic and sweat everything until translucent.

Add a little vegetable stock to everything. Now put the lentils in the pot and cook for 10 minutes, gradually adding the vegetable stock. Stir in the spices and add the coconut milk. Slice the ginger and give you soup. Let everything cook at a low temperature for about 20 minutes, stirring occasionally.

To make the soup a little thicker, briefly add the hand blender 2 - 3 times and purée the soup gently. Wash the lime warm, use the grater to grate the zest and stir into the soup.

Rinse the chili pepper and cut into fine rings. Wash off the coriander and peel off the leaves. Season the soup with salt and pepper, garnish with the coriander and the chili pepper and serve.

Quinoa In The Far East

Preparation time 40 minutes

Difficulty very easy

Servings 4 servings

Per serving

Calories 472 kcal

Protein 18 g

Fat 25 g

Carbohydrates 45 g

Ingredients

200 g quinoa

500 g broccoli(or1broccoli)

300 g oyster mushrooms

5 spring onions

4 shallots

20 g ginger (1 piece)

1 clove of garlic

2 tbsp coconut oil

1 teaspoon turmeric

1 teaspoon Indian curry powder

5 g coconut blossom sugar (1 teaspoon)

150 ml coconut milk

Salt pepper

100 g cream cheese

1 mandarin (juice)

Preparation

Wash the quinoa thoroughly in a sieve under warm running water, place in a saucepan and prepare according to the instructions on the package.

In the meantime, wash the broccoli, clean it, cut into small florets, peel off the stalk and cut into sticks. Cover and steam broccoli in a steamer basket for about 5 minutes.

In the meantime, plaster the mushrooms and cut them into bite-sized pieces. Wash and clean the spring onions and cut into rolls. Skin and chop the shallots, ginger and garlic. Bring 1 tablespoon of oil to temperature in a small saucepan and sauté shallots, ginger and garlic in it over medium heat until translucent. Add turmeric, curry powder and sugar and cook for 2 minutes until the mixture caramelizes slightly. Top up with the coconut milk and simmer for 5–8 minutes at low temperature, stirring occasionally.

Meanwhile, put the remaining oil in a pan and bring it to temperature. Sweat the mushrooms and spring onions in it at medium temperature for about 5 minutes. Add flavor to the food with salt and pepper. Put the cream cheese and mandarin juice into the curry sauce and whip the sauce until frothy using a hand blender. Season well with salt and curry powder and stir well.

Arrange the quinoa on 4 plates using the garnish rings and drape the mushroom and onion mixture and broccoli on top. Prepare the sauce decoratively on the plates and serve.

Spicy Salmon

Preparation time 30 minutes + 20 minutes

Difficulty easy

Servings 4 servings

Per serving

Calories 480 kcal

Protein 36 g

Fat 29 g

Carbohydrates 16 g

Ingredients

2 jalapeños (glass)

3 organic limes

1 tbsp chili powder

1 teaspoon brown sugar

5 ½ tbsp oil

720 g salmon fillet (4 salmon fillets)

300 g red pepper (2 red peppers)

200 g fully ripe, small mango (1 fully ripe, small mango)

1 red onion

½ bunch of coriander

Salt, pepper, sugar

150 g sour cream

Preparation

Let the jalapeños dry thoroughly in the sieve, cut in half, remove the seeds from the chilies and mash them with a fork to a fine paste. Press limes. Process the zest of one juiced lime half into zest.

In a bowl, stir the jalapeños with the chili powder, brown sugar, 2 tablespoons of oil and 2 tablespoons of lime juice and combine.

Wash the salmon fillets thoroughly, pat dry well and add to the seasoning liquid so that the fish marinates. Store in the refrigerator until further processing.

Wash the peppers, cut into four parts, separate the seeds from the pulp, wash again and place on a baking sheet with the skin facing upwards. Roast under the hot grill of the oven until the skin has turned completely black and blisters.

Then place the roasted peppers in a bowl, cover with a plate and let steam for 10 minutes.

Now peel off the black skin of the peppers and cut the peppers into fine diamonds.

Remove the peel of the mango from the fruit using a peeler. Fillet the pulp in slices from the stone and cut into diamonds.

Skin the onion and chop it very finely. Thoroughly clean the coriander and pat dry. Strip the leaves from the stem and chop them too.

In a bowl, marinate the peppers, mango, onions and coriander thoroughly with the remaining lime juice and oil (reserve 1/2 tbsp). Refine with salt, pepper and a pinch of sugar.

Stir sour cream with grated lime zest, salt and pepper until smooth.

Let a grill pan get hot and brush with the oil you have set aside. Take the salmon fillets out of the marinade and let them dry a little so that they no longer drip.

Sear them in a grill pan for 3-4 minutes on each side so that the grill pattern grills into the salmon. Put the sour cream in a piping bag and sprinkle on 4 plates using a rosette attachment, arrange 1 portion each of paprika-mango sauce and salmon fillet on top and serve.

Baked Sweet Potato With Feta, Radishes And Cress

Preparation time 60 minutes

Difficulty medium

Servings 2 servings

Per serving

Calories 563 kcal

Protein 21 g

Fat 5 g

Carbohydrates 28 g

Ingredients

2 medium sweet potatoes

200 g quark(40% fat)

50 g Greek yogurt

2 tbsp freshly squeezed lemon

100 g cucumber

5 g ginger

1 gram of garlic clove

100 g feta

1 spring onion

10 g raw radish sprouts

5raw radishes

2 tbsp olive oil

1 pinch of sea salt (fleur de sel)

1 pinch of black pepper

Preparation

Heat the oven to 200 ° C top and bottom heat. Wash the sweet potatoes and rub dry, then brush both sweet potatoes completely with oil. Place the sweet potatoes on a baking sheet lined with baking paper and bake for about 50 - 60 minutes on the middle rack.

Put the quark, yogurt and lemon juice in a bowl. Peel the garlic and immediately press it into the bowl with the garlic press. Cut off the peel of the cucumber and grate the cucumber finely. Wash and dry the spring onions and cut into thin rings. Grate the ginger and fill it with the cucumber and spring onion in the bowl, sprinkle in a little salt and pepper and whip everything creamy, if necessary add a little water if it gets too firm.

Wash the radishes and cut into thin slices. Put the sprouts in a sieve and rinse thoroughly, then dry them with a kitchen towel. Pat drily the feta cheese and crumble by hand.

Take the sweet potatoes out of the oven, notch lengthways and divide them together with the quark mixture on two plates. Scatter some feta on top and serve garnished with radishes and cress.

Tropical Vegetable Salad

Preparation time 25 minutes

Difficulty easy

Servings 4 servings

Per serving

Calories 360 kcal

Protein 3 g

Fat 25 g

Carbohydrates 25 g

Ingredients

1200 g grapefruit (4 grapefruits)

400 g ripe avocado (2 ripe avocados)

2 spring onions

2 teaspoons of cardamom pods

½ lemon

3 tbsp olive oil

2 tbsp honey

1 pinch of allspice

Salt pepper

40 g watercress (1 handful)

Preparation

Cut the grapefruit with a knife so thick that the white inner skin is also cut off.

Remove the grapefruit fillets from the separating membranes, while collecting the juice of the fruit in a bowl.

Cut the avocados in half and remove the stones from the pulp with a tablespoon. Also remove the peel from the halves of the avocados and fillet the pulp into 1 cm wide wedges.

Clean and wash the spring onions thoroughly and cut diagonally into thin rings.

Meat whole cardamom pods or the gutted cardamom seeds in a mortar. Squeeze the lemon half.

Stir grapefruit juice, 2 teaspoons of lemon juice, cardamom, oil, honey and allspice until everything has combined well. Refine the spice dressing with salt and pepper at your own discretion.

Cut out the lower thick stalks of the watercress. Cut off watercress, wash thoroughly and pat dry. Roughly chop watercress.

Mix watercress well with about 1/3 of the spice dressing. Apply the avocado fillets, spring onions, grapefruit fillets and the pickled watercress decoratively to plates. Wet with the rest of the spice dressing and enjoy immediately.

CPSIA information can be obtained
at www.ICGtesting.com
Printed in the USA
BVHW082133131221
623925BV00013B/467